Practical Manual of Clinical Obesity

Practical Manual of Clinical Obesity

Robert Kushner MD

Professor of Medicine
Northwestern University Feinberg School of Medicine
Chicago, IL, USA

Victor Lawrence MRCP PhD

Consultant Physician in Endocrinology and Diabetes Mellitus
The Arun Baksi Centre for Diabetes and Endocrinology
St Mary's Hospital
Newport, Isle of Wight, UK

Sudhesh Kumar MD FRCP FRCPath

Professor of Medicine
Warwick Medical School
University of Warwick
And Consultant Endocrinologist
University Hospitals Coventry and Warwickshire
Coventry, UK

WILEY-BLACKWELL

A John Wiley & Sons, Ltd., Publication

Contents

Contents

Preface

According to the World Health Organization (WHO), obesity is one of the greatest public health challenges of the 21st century. In 2008, more than 1.4 billion adults, 20 years and older, were found to be overweight. Of these, over 200 million men and nearly 300 million women were obese. In the 27 member states of the European Union, approximately 60% of adults and over 20% of school-age children are overweight or obese. The prevalence of overweight and obesity in the USA is even more distressing, affecting over 68% of adults and 33% of children and adolescents. Overweight and obesity are now linked to more deaths worldwide than underweight. The cause for the rapid increase in the prevalence of obesity is multifaceted, brought about by an interaction between predisposing genetic and metabolic factors and a rapidly changing "modern" environment.

The health risks of excess weight have been demonstrated in multiple population studies. Obesity significantly increases a person's risk of developing numerous non-communicable diseases (NCDs), including cardiovascular disease, cancer, diabetes, sleep disturbance, and other disabilities. The risk of developing more than one of these diseases (co-morbidity) also increases with increasing body weight. Accordingly, obesity-related health-care costs are soaring and contribute to an increasing percentage of total health-care expenditures. These data suggest that halting and reversing the obesity epidemic will require involvement of multiple stakeholders, including the medical profession.

Regardless of which health-care area a provider is working, clinicians are being called upon to provide care for persons affected by obesity. It is no longer sufficient to simply advise our patients to "eat less and move more." Obesity is now considered a complex disease determined by genetic, physiological, behavioral, psychosocial, cultural, economic, and societal factors. The etiological mechanisms underlying obesity-related co-morbidities, for example, hemodynamic alterations, insulin resistance, hormonal abnormalities, ectopic fat, and secretion of adipokines, continue to be clarified. Research over the past decade has also elucidated the metabolic and genetic control systems that govern regulation of body weight and energy expenditure, leading to the development of novel pharmacological and surgical interventions. Each year new intervention trials demonstrate the beneficial effect of weight loss on a myriad of obesity-related co-morbidities.

In an effort to translate the emerging science and practice of obesity care for clinicians, the *Practical Manual of Clinical Obesity* has been written as a practical, evidence-based companion guide to the textbook *Clinical Obesity in Adults and Children*, edited by P.G. Kopelman, I.D. Caterson, and W.H. Dietz. The manual is intended for physicians, nurses, allied health professionals, and students who care for overweight and obese individuals. The 20 concise chapters of the manual are divided into three major sections: The Biology of Obesity—Why It Occurs, Clinical Management of the Obese Individual, and Clinical Management of Obesity-Related Co-morbidities. Each chapter includes features that are directly intended to improve its readability and usefulness for the busy clinician—key points, case studies, boxed figures, pitfalls, key web links, and references. A collective effort has been made by the three editors to write all chapters with "one voice." We hope that we have succeeded in publishing a manual that will be a valuable resource for the care of patients affected by obesity.

R.F. Kushner
V. Lawrence
S. Kumar

PART 1

The Biology of Obesity—Why It Occurs

Victor Lawrence, Section Editor

CHAPTER 1

Energy Balance and Body Weight Homeostasis

Key points
- Energy intake is highly variable, and mechanisms to defend a "set point" in energy stores appear to have evolved.
- Energy is spent doing useful physical, chemical, and electrical work and also producing heat (thermogenesis) as a by-product of these activities.
- Thermogenesis is subject to regulation and may be adapted to prevailing energy balance.
- Basal metabolic rate (BMR) increases predominantly in proportion to lean body mass and is higher in the obese. Its fall with caloric restriction may present a barrier to long-term weight loss.
- Energy is also spent in voluntary (exercise) and other non-exercise activity thermogenesis (NEAT).
- Spontaneous physical activity (SPA) is a major component of NEAT and is regulated by the sympathetic nervous system (SNS), and its fall with caloric restriction may present a barrier to successful weight loss.
- Genetic and acquired variations in the amount and efficiency of these largely unconscious processes may explain some inter- and intra-individual variability in energy metabolism and thus predisposition toward obesity.
- Food (energy) intake is subject to complex regulation by circulating and gut-derived signals which include leptin.
- In addition to its effects on energy intake, leptin has the ability to stimulate adaptive thermogenesis via SPA, uncoupling of oxidative phosphorylation, and possibly via futile cycling. Many of these effects depend on the SNS.
- Leptin deficiency or receptor mutations are a very rare cause of human obesity. Nevertheless, relative defects in leptin action may (at least in theory) influence body weight homeostasis and are the subject of current research.
- Brown adipose tissue (BAT) exists in adults; it is regulated by the SNS and contributes to thermogenesis. Stimulating its differentiation and activation is a target of current research.

Practical Manual of Clinical Obesity, First Edition. Robert Kushner, Victor Lawrence and Sudhesh Kumar.

CASE STUDIES

Case study 1

CF is a 24-year-old woman with a body mass index (BMI) of 32 kg/m². She describes an apparently healthy diet which she considers to be no higher in calories than that taken by many of her friends and family who do not have weight problems. She also walks regularly. She feels immensely frustrated over her seeming inability to achieve or maintain an ideal body weight despite good habits and is starting to feel like giving up.

Comment: You explore her concerns and find that she is certain that she has an undiagnosed metabolic problem leading to a slow metabolism, a problem she feels runs in her family despite repeatedly normal tests of thyroid function. You explain that the body does adapt over time to a change in weight and the new higher or lower weight tends to be opposed by changes in metabolic rate and overall energy expenditure which can make the achievement and maintenance of weight loss progressively harder. You arrange to measure her resting metabolic rate principally to demonstrate to her that it lies in the range expected for body composition, age, and sex. You explain how SPA may lessen over time in people who are losing weight and discuss ways of maintaining this, for example, walking to the shops, taking stairs rather than escalators, and measuring the number of daily footsteps with a pedometer. You also explain that periods of weight maintenance are perfectly logical (and successful) as part of a long-term program of weight control and may permit the body to acclimatize and form a new set point—the only outcome that represents failure is to give up and regain any weight lost. She finds sufficient motivation in these concepts to re-energize herself in her weight loss goals.

Case study 2

LW, an obese 58-year-old man, has been very gradually but successfully reducing his weight with your support over the past year. However, his weight loss trajectory has stopped over the past month and he has begun to regain weight.

Comment: You enquire about changes in his circumstances and discover that his primary care physician recently started him on a beta-blocker following possible, although incompletely ascertained, intolerance of first-line drug therapy for his hypertension. You explain that beta-blockers inhibit the actions of the SNS. This could affect his overall energy balance in several ways, including reduced lipolysis (and possibly therefore reduced futile cycling of fatty acids between free and esterified forms) and reductions in thermogenesis, SPA, and in overall metabolic rate. Furthermore, beta-blockers may also reduce exercise capacity and cause fatigue, all of which may counter attempted weight loss. Although the magnitude of these effects is small (typically 1–2 kg, 2.2–4.4 lb), it is possible that some individuals may be affected more than this. Older "non-selective" beta-blockers appear to be more problematic than newer "cardioselective" agents. On discussing this, together with possible adverse effects on insulin sensitivity, you agree to try an angiotensin receptor blocking agent.

Introduction

In most individuals, body weight remains relatively stable over years to decades despite wide variations in energy intake and expenditure. This would seem to suggest that body weight is rigorously defended by homeostatic mechanisms. However, whilst a useful defense against the development of obesity, any tendency to defend a set point once obesity is established may act as a barrier to the achievement and maintenance of planned weight loss.

Many individuals seeking professional help in relation to their own obesity become confused or frustrated by what appears to be inability to lose weight (or a tendency to gain weight) despite behaviors that might appear no less healthy than other individuals who do not appear to have a weight problem. Some will have developed counterproductive health beliefs that may act as barriers to weight loss (e.g., that they must have a slow metabolism and that this is genetically programmed or is the result of some undiagnosed metabolic disorder and therefore beyond their control). These misunderstandings can rapidly evolve into a sense of "learned helplessness" and all too often result in disengagement and failure to achieve goals.

Clear and accurate explanations of the complexities of energy balance regulation are often of practical help, particularly where such frustration or despondency exists.

Basic concepts and principles in human energetics

Energy balance and laws of thermodynamics

According to the *first law of thermodynamics*,

Energy intake = Energy expenditure + Change (Δ) in energy stores

The chemical energy obtained from food is used to perform a variety of work, such as

- synthesis of new macromolecules (*chemical work*)
- muscular contraction (*mechanical work*)
- maintenance of ionic gradients across membranes (*electrical work*)

Thus, if the total energy contained in the body (in the form of fat, protein, and glycogen) of a given individual is not altered (i.e., Δ energy stores=0), then energy expenditure must be equal to energy intake and the individual is said to be in a state of *energy balance*.

If the intake and expenditure of energy are not equal, then a change in body energy content will occur, with *negative energy balance* resulting in the degradation of the body's energy stores (glycogen, fat, and protein) or *positive energy balance* resulting in an increase in body energy stores, primarily as fat.

The *second law of thermodynamics* makes a distinction between the potential energy of food, useful work, and heat. It states essentially that

Energy expenditure = Work done + Heat generated

and describes the fact that when food is utilized in the body, these processes must be accompanied inevitably by some loss of heat. In other words, the conversion of available food energy is not a perfectly efficient process: about

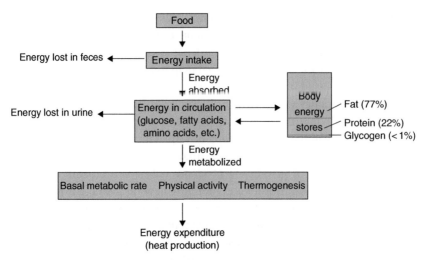

Figure 1.1 Principles of energy balance within a schematic framework that depicts the transformation of energy from food to heat throughout the body. Note that on diets typically consumed in developed countries, the total energy losses in feces and urine are small (about 5%) so that the metabolizable energy available from these diets is around 95%. Reproduced from Kopelman *et al.* (eds). *Clinical Obesity in Adults and Children*, 3rd edn, Blackwell Publishing, Oxford, 2010, with permission from Blackwell Publishing.

75% of the chemical energy contained in foods may be ultimately dissipated as heat because of the inefficiency of intermediary metabolism. The energy "wasted" as heat may be calculated as the sum of BMR and adaptive thermogenesis. Adaptive thermogenesis refers to the increase in resting energy expenditure in response to stimuli such as food intake, cold, stress, and drugs.

Components of energy expenditure

It is customary to consider human energy expenditure as being made up of three components:
- Energy spent on basal metabolism (BMR)
- Energy spent on physical activity (work done plus exercise- or non-exercise-associated thermogenesis)
- The increase in resting energy expenditure in response to stimuli such as food, cold, stress, and drugs (adaptive thermogenesis).

These three components are depicted in Figure 1.1 and are described in the following text.

Basal (or resting) metabolic rate (BMR)

This is the largest component of energy expenditure for most individuals. Typically, BMR accounts for 60–75% of daily energy expenditure. It is measured under standardized conditions, that is, in an awake subject lying in the supine position, in a state of physical and mental rest in a comfortable warm environment, and in the morning in the post-absorptive state, usually 10–12 h after the last meal.

By far the most important determinant of BMR is body size, in particular lean (fat-free) body mass which is influenced by weight, height, age, and gender. Lean body mass is increased in obese individuals, although to a lesser extent than fat mass. This means that, counter to many obese subject's expectations, their BMR is almost certainly higher than that of their lean counterparts, and a low BMR is, with the debatable exception of hypothyroidism, virtually never a direct cause of obesity. On the contrary, a higher BMR in obese subjects tends to oppose further weight gain, although its fall with weight loss may act as a barrier to successful weight management.

Measurement of BMR by indirect calorimetry is a non-invasive test used in a number of obesity clinics often as a means of demonstrating to an individual that their BMR lies within the range expected for body composition, age, and sex.

In addition to increasing BMR, there appears to be a decrease in metabolic efficiency in obese subjects, which also acts to favor a return to the previous "set point." Subjects made under experimental conditions to maintain body weight at a level 10% above their initial body weight show a compensatory change in resting energy expenditure (approximately 15%), which reflects changes in metabolic efficiency that oppose the maintenance of a body weight that is above or below the set or preferred body weight.

Energy expenditure due to physical activity

Physical activity can represent up to 70% of daily energy expenditure in an individual involved in heavy manual work or competition athletics, although values of 10–25% are more usual in modern Westernized civilizations.

Energy expended in physical activity may be thought of as being spent either on deliberate "exercise" or on all other "non-exercise" activities. Non-exercise activities may be deliberate and consciously modifiable (e.g., daily tasks such as work, shopping, cooking), may be related to posture and balance, or may be involuntary purposeless movements (e.g., fidgeting, movements during sleep), the latter being termed spontaneous physical activity (SPA). The energy dissipated as heat through such forms of "non-exercise" activities is called non-exercise activity thermogenesis (NEAT).

Levels of SPA are regulated in part by the SNS. Losses in body weight are accompanied by a major reduction in SPA, which can persist for several months after weight recovery and favor disproportionate recovery of fat mass. Twenty-four-hour energy expenditure attributed to SPA may vary between 100 and 700 kcal/day between individuals and can predict subsequent weight gain after a period of caloric restriction. In one study, more than 60% of the increase in total daily energy expenditure in response to overfeeding could be attributed to SPA, variability of which was the best predictor of individual weight gain.

Other components of NEAT also differ between obese and lean individuals. One study showed that obese participants were seated, on average, for 2 h longer per day than lean participants. This difference (corresponding to about 350 kcal/day) was not altered after weight gain in lean individuals or weight loss in obese individuals, suggesting that it might be biologically determined. Increased skeletal muscle work efficiency after experimentally induced weight loss has also been reported.

It seems likely that such mechanisms form a barrier to the effectiveness of planned weight loss regimens and are subject to as yet largely unknown genetic influences.

Energy expenditure in response to various thermogenic stimuli

Exertion, whether as exercise or as NEAT, generates heat as a by-product and contributes to thermogenesis. However, several non-exertional thermogenic stimuli with relevance to body weight regulation also exist. These include the following.

Diet-induced thermogenesis or the "thermic effect of food"

The thermic effect of food refers to heat production due to the mechanical and chemical consequences of food ingestion. This process dissipates some 7–9% of the energy content of a typical mixed meal and is affected by meal size, meal composition, meal frequency, thermogenic ingredients such as caffeine, and the individual subject's insulin sensitivity.

Psychological thermogenesis

Psychological thermogenesis refers to heat dissipation over baseline in response to states such as anxiety or stress. Thermogenesis in this setting may depend on both changes in physical activity (e.g., SPA) and via central (e.g., endocrine) mechanisms.

Cold-induced thermogenesis

Energy is spent on maintaining temperature homeostasis through "shivering" (muscular activity) and "non-shivering" (SNS activity, partly via BAT) responses to cold. The extent to which maintenance of warm environments through modern central heating may contribute to obesity is at present unknown, although average temperature settings continue to rise steadily and there is some evidence that a lack of need to respond to "mild thermogenic stress" may lead to a long-term loss of BAT.

Drug-induced thermogenesis

Caffeine, alcohol, nicotine, and other prescription or "recreational" drugs may stimulate the dissipation of energy as heat. Of these, the most clinically relevant is probably the effect of smoking cessation on body weight with some 7 kg (15.4 lb) weight gained on average, partly through changes in food intake and partly through a reduction in thermogenesis. Discouraging the abuse of tobacco for weight control purposes remains a considerable practical challenge for clinicians.

Mechanisms of thermogenesis

The SNS, through its neurotransmitter norepinephrine (NE), acts via α- and β-adrenoceptors to influence heat production by either increasing the use of ATP (e.g., ion pumping and substrate cycling) or by reducing the efficiency of ATP synthesis. These actions induce metabolic inefficiency, which has the potential to oppose any change from the body weight set point.

The recent realization that brown fat exists in adult humans has rekindled interest in pharmacologic activation of BAT in anti-obesity therapy.

Leptin is a cytokine whose principal role is thought to be to defend minimum fat stores in the longer term. As fat stores fall, leptin levels also fall, with the net result being that of reduced thermogenesis and increased metabolic efficiency. This action is an example of a "lipostatic" model of weight defense: the set point is for body fat stores, and homeostatic regulation (e.g., by leptin pathways) acts to defend this set point (Box 1.1).

Inter-individual variability in metabolic adaptation

A striking feature of virtually all experiments of human overfeeding (lasting from a few weeks to a few months) is the wide range of individual variability in the amount of weight gain per unit of excess energy consumed. Some of

---

Box 1.1 Leptin effects on thermogenesis.

Diminished skeletal muscle work efficiency

Increased SPA

Thermogenic action of leptin via the SNS on BAT and skeletal muscle

Central effects on SPA-associated thermogenesis

Regulation of reward signals, motivated behaviors that influence appetite, and locomotor activity

Direct action on skeletal muscle, possibly through stimulation of "futile" substrate cycling between *de novo* lipogenesis and lipid oxidation

these differences in the efficiency of weight gain could be attributed to inter-individual variability in the gain of lean tissue relative to fat tissue (i.e., variability in the composition of weight gain), but mostly lie in the ability to convert excess calories to heat, that is, in the large inter-individual capacity for diet-induced (and other forms of adaptive) thermogenesis.

Over- and under-feeding experiments suggest that in addition to the control of food intake, changes in the composition of weight (via partitioning between lean and fat tissues) and in metabolic efficiency (via adaptive thermogenesis) both play an important role in the regulation of body weight and body composition. Evidence from identical-twin studies suggests that the magnitude of these adaptive changes is strongly influenced by the genetic makeup of the individual.

Current evidence suggests the existence of two distinct but overlapping control systems underlying adaptive thermogenesis.

One control system responds rapidly to attenuate the impact of changes in food intake on changes in body weight through alterations in the activity of the SNS which is suppressed during starvation and increased during overfeeding.

The other control system, exemplified by leptin, has a slower time-constant since it operates as a feedback loop between the size of the fat stores and thermogenesis. Its suppression during weight (and fat) losses serves to restore body fat to its set or preferred level.

These autoregulatory control systems operating through adjustments in heat production or thermogenesis play a crucial role in attenuating and correcting deviations of body weight from its set or preferred value. The extent to which these adjustments through adaptive thermogenesis are brought about is dependent upon the environment (e.g., diet composition) and is highly variable from one individual to another. In societies where food is plentiful all year round and physical activity demands are low, the resultant subtle variations among individuals in adaptive thermogenesis can, in dynamic systems and over the long term, be important in determining long-term constancy of body weight in some and in provoking the drift toward obesity in others.

Pitfalls

- Significant weight loss is followed by metabolic adaptation which tends to oppose it. This includes reduced SPA, increased metabolic efficiency, reduced resting metabolic rate, and increased skeletal work efficiency. Losing weight in the short term is often achievable with relative ease. Difficulties presented by defense of a set point are a common reason for failure to maintain weight loss in the longer term, and explanations may help keep the patient engaged.
- Metabolic rate is higher in the obese and correlates best with lean body mass which is also higher in them. However, many obese people consider that they have an

undiagnosed metabolic problem and may lose confidence if this belief is not sympathetically addressed.
- Energy may be spent by increasing NEAT, for example, taking stairs, not using a car to travel short distances, cycling to work, and so on.
- Periods of weight maintenance may be an effective strategy to permit adaptation to a newly reduced body weight and is certainly better than giving up. The only completely failed weight loss episode is one where weight is initially lost but regained after despondency sets in, the episode concluding with acquisition of a new weight higher than that at the start.
- Not exploring a patient's belief that because they find weight loss harder than others, they are unable to do it. There is no doubt that some people and some lifestyles do present challenges, but they can be overcome.
- Diets that are difficult to digest, require energy to obtain and chew, and that are low in calorie density may help with weight loss. Compare, for example, walking to a market to buy fresh carrots or growing one's own (and perhaps eating them raw) with snacking on crisps or biscuits kept in the house.
- Not appreciating sympathetically the degree to which the thermogenic and appetite-reducing effects of tobacco consumption may be used by some patients as an adjunct to weight control.

Key web links

Weight Control Information Network (National Institute of Diabetes and Digestive and Kidney Diseases). http://win.niddk.nih.gov/resources/ [accessed on December 29, 2012].
Association for the Study of Obesity. http://www.aso.org.uk/ [accessed on December 29, 2012].
National Institutes of Health. http://health.nih.gov/topic/Obesity [accessed on December 29, 2012].

Further reading

Garland, T., Jr., Schutz, H., Chappell, M.A. *et al.* (2011) The biological control of voluntary exercise, spontaneous physical activity and daily energy expenditure in relation to obesity: Human and rodent perspectives. *Journal Experimental Biology*, 214 (Pt 2), 206–229.
Gautron, L. & Elmquist, J.K. (2011) Sixteen years and counting: An update on leptin in energy balance. *Journal of Clinical Investigation*, 121, 2087–2093.
King, N.A., Hopkins, M., Caudwell, P., Stubbs, R.J. & Blundell J.E. (2008) Individual variability following 12 weeks of supervised exercise: Identification and characterization of compensation for exercise-induced weight loss. *International Journal of Obesity*, 32, 177–184.
Li, M.D. (2011) Leptin and beyond: An odyssey to the central control of body weight. *Yale Journal of Biology and Medicine*, 84, 1–7.
van Marken Lichtenbelt, W.D. & Schrauwen, P. (2011) Implications of nonshivering thermogenesis for energy balance regulation in humans. *American Journal of Physiology – Regulatory Integrative and Comparative Physiology*, 301, R285–R296.

van Marken Lichtenbelt, W.D., Vanhommerig, J.W., Smulders, N.M. *et al.* (2009) Cold-activated brown adipose tissue in healthy men. *New England Journal of Medicine*, 360, 1500–1508. Erratum in *New England Journal of Medicine* (2009), 360, 1917.

Richard, D. & Picard, F. (2011) Brown fat biology and thermogenesis. *Frontiers in Bioscience*, 16, 1233–1260.

Rosenbaum, M., Hirsch, J., Gallagher, D.A. & Leibel, R.L. (2008) Long-term persistence of adaptive thermogenesis in subjects who have maintained a reduced body weight. *American Journal of Clinical Nutrition*, 88, 906–912.

Schoeller, D.A. (2009) The energy balance equation: Looking back and looking forward are two very different views. *Nutrition Review*, 67, 249–254.

Sharma, A.M., Pischon, T., Hardt, S., Kunz, I. & Luft, F.C. (2001) Hypothesis: ß-adrenergic receptor blockers and weight gain—a systematic analysis. *Hypertension*, 37, 250–254.

CHAPTER 2

The Genetic Basis of Obesity

Key points

- Genetic influences may explain up to 70% of population variation in BMI. However, the influence of very many genes, all interacting with the environment, is likely to determine individual susceptibility. The presence of risk alleles in all the currently known susceptibility loci only explains a few percent of this variance.
- Most genetic influences are likely to be polygenic (depending on very many different genes rather than a single risk allele).
- Complex gene–environment interactions are likely to explain why obesity has become so prevalent recently, although the human gene pool has changed little over the past 30 years. This is well exemplified by the fat mass and obesity-associated gene (*FTO*) risk allele.
- Many genetic forms of obesity are syndromic: the presence of learning difficulties, growth disorders, dysmorphic features, or profound early-onset obesity should certainly prompt consideration of a syndromic form of obesity.
- A number of monogenic obesity syndromes have now been described, most notably that of leptin deficiency but also including MC4 receptor and pro-opiomelanocortin (POMC) mutations among others. The rarity of these conditions means that their importance lies more in unraveling mechanisms and pathways important in obesity rather than in the clinical management of the individual patient. Nevertheless, profound early-onset obesity, particularly if associated with other specific features, for example, adrenocortical insufficiency, recurrent infection, and a family history of hypogonadotropic hypogonadism, should prompt consideration of these rare but potentially treatable monogenic syndromes.
- MC4 receptor mutations may explain up to 6% of non-syndromic early-onset severe obesity, although the precise role of risk alleles in more typical obesity is currently debated.
- Unraveling genetic mechanisms has done much to further the understanding of regulatory pathways governing body weight and perhaps how we have come to view the whole problem of obesity.
- Further advances in obesity genetics have the potential to herald the development of more rational mechanism-based interventions at both the individual and population levels.

Practical Manual of Clinical Obesity, First Edition. Robert Kushner, Victor Lawrence and Sudhesh Kumar.
© 2013 John Wiley & Sons, Ltd. Published 2013 by John Wiley & Sons, Ltd.

CASE STUDIES

Case study 1

A 42-year-old woman who, together with several other members of her family, has been struggling with her obesity for some years has heard that between 40% and 70% of adult obesity may be attributable to genetic constitution. She has essentially given up on trying to lose weight as a consequence and is referred to you for advice. She asks what can be done about her genetic problem and how long it will take to find a cure.

Comment: You acknowledge her feelings of negativity, examine her to exclude features of monogenetic or syndromic obesity, and explain that although overall genetic influences do appear to be important and are the subject of much research interest, no one single gene is likely to be responsible in her case. You go on to explain that any one individual's personal energy balance equation depends on the sum of the tiny effects of hundreds or possibly thousands of genes, none of which alter the fact that she will lose weight if she is able to achieve a state of negative energy balance through diet and exercise. Genetic influences leading to the "thrifty phenotype" may well explain why some people have to work harder to achieve and maintain weight loss than others but do not make it impossible to do so. You explain how genes will have changed little over the past 50 years and it is the effect of our changed environment on these genes that has led to the recent upsurge in obesity and we do have some control over our environment. You therefore encourage her to plan small but achievable lifestyle changes that she agrees she can adopt. You point out that genetic studies may well identify useful treatments for obesity in the future, although it usually takes many years for a novel drug to come to the market from its first conception.

Case study 2

A 34-year-old man with a BMI of 46 kg/m², new onset type 2 diabetes (T2DM), and hypertension has undertaken several professionally supported weight management programs over the past few years with little or no sustained success. He had severe early-onset obesity and took part in a clinical study during which he was found to be a heterozygous carrier of an MC4 receptor mutation known to be associated with obesity. He asks whether you think that he might benefit from bariatric surgery or whether the known genetic problem means that he should wait for a cure.

Comment: You acknowledge that this is a difficult decision for him. However, the time frame for specific treatments to come into routine clinical use is long and there would be no guarantee that such treatment would work, at least before significant harm may have accrued to him through his obesity-related co-morbidities, particularly diabetes. In the meantime, he has not been able to reverse his obesity despite appropriate interventions, and the development of diabetes and hypertension make bariatric surgery a serious option for him to consider. You explain that although there are few data, the expected effect of his genetic constitution would be to impair satiety, which could at least theoretically (and, in one study, has been shown to) lead to complications of laparoscopic gastric banding. This, together with the favorable endocrine effects of bypass surgery (particularly in the setting of T2DM), might favor this type of procedure which has been shown in at least one small study to be no less effective in heterozygous carriers of an MC4 receptor than in unaffected subjects. You agree to make a referral for consideration of Roux-en-Y gastric bypass (RYGB).

Introduction

Much emphasis from a public health perspective has been rightly focused on the concept of the "obesogenic" environment, and there is little doubt that post-industrial and other changes have contributed to this over recent decades. However, not all individuals exposed to this environment develop obesity. This leads to the concept that, in most cases at least, it is likely to be a combination of an obesogenic environment and genetic predisposition that leads to the expression of clinical obesity. Put another way, the large changes in energy consumption and expenditure over recent decades may be seen as having provided the opportunity for predisposed individuals to become obese. Twin and other studies have led to a widely accepted estimate that 40–70% of observed variation in BMI has a genetic basis. Current insight into the genetic basis of obesity has come from the study of

1 candidate genes—genes that are known to encode proteins involved in the regulation of energy intake or expenditure (e.g., β3-adrenoceptor involved in energy expenditure, melanocortin-4 receptor (MC4R) involved in appetite regulation)

2 genetic syndromes in which obesity is a feature (e.g., Prader–Willi syndrome (PWS))

3 rare forms of monogenic (single-gene) obesity without other syndromic features, for example, *ob/ob* mouse, leptin-deficient humans, and POMC gene mutations

4 genome-wide associations in large heterogeneous populations

In the last 10 years, seven single-gene defects causing severe human obesity have been identified. Over 30 genetic syndromes of which obesity forms a part are also described. Studies of patients with mutations in these molecules have shed light on the physiology of body weight regulation in humans—indeed, the discovery of leptin from studies of the genetically obese *ob/ob* mouse was to revolutionize the whole field of obesity research.

Many individuals with obesity consider the possibility that they may have some undiagnosed metabolic derangement, possibly with a genetic basis, which, if characterized, would reduce their predisposition to maintaining a state of positive energy balance. Thus, a knowledge of current concepts in the genetics of obesity is important for those seeking to advise patients affected by, or at risk from, obesity and is the focus of this chapter.

Evidence for the heritability of fat mass

There is considerable evidence to suggest that, like height, weight is a heritable trait.

Adoption studies

Adoption studies are useful in separating the common environmental effects since adoptive parents and their adoptive offspring share only environmental sources of variance, while the adoptees and their biological parents share only genetic sources of variance. One of the largest series, based on over 5000 subjects from the Danish adoption register, showed a strong relationship between the BMI of adoptees and biological parents across the whole range of body fatness but none when compared with the adoptive parents.

Twin studies

Monozygotic co-twins share 100% of their genes, and dizygotes, 50% on average. Heritability estimates the contribution of genetic influence by comparing the similarity of a trait within monozygotic twins with the similarity within dizygotic twins making the assumption of a similar shared environment. Genetic contribution to the BMI in these studies has been estimated to be in the region of 64–84%.

The most powerful tool for estimating genetic influence is the study of monozygotic twins reared apart, which has all the advantages of a twin study but does not rely on the assumption of identical environmental exposure. Correlation of monozygotic twins reared apart is virtually a direct estimate of the heritability, although monozygotic twins do share the intra-uterine environment, which may contribute to lasting differences in body mass in later life. Estimates of obesity heritability in these studies vary from 40% to 70%, depending on age at separation of twins and the length of follow-up.

Familial resemblance in nutrient intake has been reported in parents and their children, although the extent to which this is genetically determined is unclear. Twin data suggest that there are notable genetic influences on the overall intake of nutrients, size and frequency of meals, and intake of particular foods. Approximately 40% of the variance in resting metabolic rate, thermic effect of food, and energy cost of low- to moderate-intensity exercise may be explained by inherited characteristics. In addition, significant familial resemblance for level of habitual physical activity has been reported in a large cohort of healthy female twins.

Gene–environment interactions

The gene pool is unlikely to have changed substantially over the past 50–100 years, whereas the environment has changed markedly. If genetic influences are as important as is suggested by estimates of heritability, then it is likely that genes rely on environmental triggers (e.g., sedentary lifestyle, constant availability of calorie-dense foods) for their expression. Pima Indians, for example, living in the USA are on average 25 kg heavier than Pima Indians living in Mexico, and the difference is likely to be due to gene–environment interactions. This effect is also seen in overfeeding or under-feeding experiments, where differences in metabolic adaptation between individuals to the same environmental stress (e.g., in weight change, metabolic rate, compensatory effects on physical activity, hunger scores) are likely to have a genetic basis.

Molecular mechanisms involved in energy homeostasis

Rodent models of obesity

Since the early 1900s, a number of obese inbred strains of mice, both dominant (yellow, *Ay/a*) and recessive (*ob/ob, db/db, fa/fa, tb/tb*), have been studied. In the 1990s, the genes responsible for these syndromes were identified, and these observations have given substantial insights into the physiological disturbances that can lead to obesity, the metabolic and endocrine abnormalities associated with the obese phenotype, and the more detailed anatomic and neurochemical pathways that regulate energy intake and energy expenditure. These studies provide the basic framework upon which the understanding of the more complex mechanisms in humans can be built.

Leptin–melanocortin pathway

The initial observations in this field were made as a result of positional cloning strategies in two strains of severely obese mice. Severely obese *ob/ob* mice were found to harbor mutations in the *ob* gene, resulting in a complete lack of its protein product, leptin. Administration of recombinant leptin reduced the food intake and body weight of leptin-deficient *ob/ob* mice and corrected all their neuro-endocrine and metabolic abnormalities. The signaling form of the leptin receptor is deleted in *db/db* mice, which are consequently unresponsive to endogenous or exogenous leptin. The identification of these two proteins established the first components of a nutritional feedback loop from adipose tissue to the brain. However, it is considered that the physiological role of leptin in humans and rodents might be to act as a signal for starvation, because as fat mass increases, further rises in leptin have a limited ability to suppress food intake and prevent obesity.

Considerable attention has been focused on deciphering the hypothalamic pathways that co-ordinate the behavioral and metabolic effects downstream of leptin. The first-order neuronal targets of leptin action in the brain are anorectic (reducing food intake) POMC and orexigenic (increasing food intake) neuropeptide-Y/agouti-related protein (NPY/AgRP) neurons in the hypothalamic arcuate nucleus. POMC is sequentially cleaved by prohormone convertases to yield peptides including α-melanocyte-stimulating hormone (MSH) that acts as a suppressor of feeding behavior, probably through MC4R. In fact, targeted disruption of MC4R in rodents leads to increased food intake, obesity, severe early-onset hyperinsulinemia, and increased linear growth; heterozygotes have an intermediate phenotype compared to homozygotes and wild-type mice.

Human monogenic obesity syndromes

Congenital leptin deficiency

In 1997, two severely obese cousins from a highly consanguineous family of Pakistani origin were reported. Both children had undetectable levels of serum leptin and were found to be homozygous for a frameshift mutation in the *ob* gene (ΔG133), which resulted in a truncated protein that was not secreted. A few other families with broadly similar features have subsequently been reported from other regions.

Affected subjects are characterized by severe early-onset obesity and intense hyperphagia with food-seeking behavior and an inability to discriminate between appetizing and bland foods. Hyperinsulinemia, hypogonadotropic hypogonadism, and an advanced bone age are also common features. Children with leptin deficiency have profound abnormalities of T-cell number and function, consistent with high rates of childhood infection and a high reported rate of childhood mortality from infection.

Response to leptin therapy

Dramatic and beneficial effects of daily subcutaneous injections of leptin in reducing body weight and fat mass in three congenitally leptin-deficient children were first reported in 2002. All children showed a response to initial leptin doses designed to produce plasma leptin levels at only 10% of those predicted by height and weight. The most dramatic example of leptin effects was with a 3-year-old boy, severely disabled by gross obesity (wt 42 kg), who weighed only 32 kg (75th centile for weight) after 48 months of leptin therapy (Figure 2.1).

Partial leptin deficiency

The major question with respect to the potential therapeutic use of leptin in more common forms of obesity relates to the shape of the leptin dose–response curve. Raising leptin levels from undetectable to detectable has

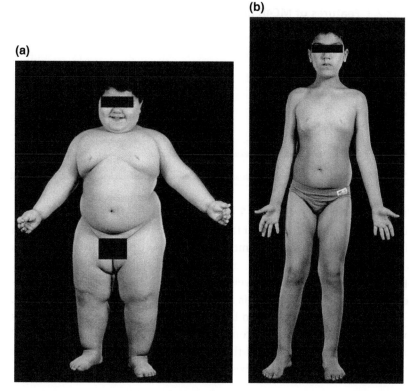

Figure 2.1 Human male (a) before and (b) after leptin treatment. Reproduced from Kopelman *et al.* (eds) (2010) *Clinical Obesity in Adults and Children*, 3rd edn, Blackwell Publishing, Oxford, with permission from Blackwell Publishing.

profound effects on appetite and weight, but the administration of supraphysiological doses has little useful effect as most obese individuals already have leptin levels well above the dose–response curve. Whether or not enhancing transport of leptin into the central nervous system (CNS), where it has its major effects, could improve the therapeutic prospects for leptin is at present unknown.

POMC deficiency

Several unrelated obese children with homozygous or compound heterozygous mutations in POMC have been reported. These children are hyperphagic, developing early-onset obesity as a result of impaired melanocortin signaling in the hypothalamus. They present in neonatal life with adrenal crisis due to isolated adrenocorticotropic hormone (ACTH) deficiency (POMC is a precursor of ACTH in the pituitary) and have pale skin and red hair due to the lack of MSH function in melanocortin-1 receptors in the skin.

Box 2.1 Features of MC4R mutation.

- Common
- Non-syndromic
- Inheritance complex
- High growth velocity
- Increased final height
- Insulin resistance
- Increased bone mineral density
- Increased lean body mass

Prohormone convertase 1 deficiency

Further evidence for the role of the melanocortin system in the regulation of body weight in humans comes from the description of three patients with severe childhood obesity, abnormal glucose homeostasis, very low plasma insulin but elevated levels of proinsulin, hypogonadotropic hypogonadism, and hypocortisolemia associated with elevated levels of POMC.

These subjects were found to be compound heterozygous/homozygous for mutations in prohormone convertase 1, and its failure to cleave POMC to generate α-MSH, a ligand of the anorexigenic MC4R, is likely to be the predominant mechanism for obesity in these patients.

MC4R deficiency

Mutations in MC4R have been reported in up to 6% of patients with severe early-onset obesity and are found at a frequency of approximately 1 in 1000 in the general UK population, making this one of the most common human monogenic diseases.

Detailed phenotypic studies of patients with MC4R mutations reveal that this syndrome is characterized by an increase in lean body mass and bone mineral density, a marked increase in linear growth throughout childhood, hyperphagia, and severe hyperinsulinemia. These features are similar to those seen in MC4R knockout mice, suggesting the preservation of the relevant melanocortin pathways between rodents and humans. Of particular note is the finding that the severity of receptor dysfunction seen in *in vitro* assays can predict the amount of food ingested at a test meal by the subject harboring that particular mutation (Box 2.1).

Fat mass and obesity-associated gene (*FTO*)

FTO was among the genes highlighted in several genome-wide association studies for type 2 diabetes mellitus (T2DM), but the effect on diabetes has subsequently been shown to be mediated via increased BMI. Individuals with one copy of the "risk allele" are 1.67 times more likely to be obese than those with no affected alleles and have a mean excess body weight of approximately 3–4 kg. Homozygous individuals with two copies of the risk allele are as much as 2.67 times more likely to be obese than those with no copies. The effect of this gene appears to be primarily expressed by means of increased energy intake rather than by reduced energy expenditure, and at least one study has shown a gene–environment interaction predisposing carriers of *FTO* risk alleles to a greater propensity for gaining weight in conditions of low physical activity and high dietary fat intake than control subjects. Furthermore, homozygotes were found in one study to be less successful in weight loss than unaffected counterparts.

Pleiotropic ("syndromic") obesity

It is well established that obesity runs in families, although the vast majority of cases do not segregate with a clear Mendelian pattern of inheritance. There are about 30 Mendelian disorders with obesity as a clinical feature but often associated with mental retardation, dysmorphic features, and organ-specific developmental abnormalities. The commonest of these (estimated prevalence 1:25,000) is PWS, which is characterized by obesity, hypotonia, mental retardation, short stature, hypogonadotropic hypogonadism, and small hands and feet. Some of the other syndromic forms of obesity are listed in Table 2.1.

Summary

Genetic factors are likely to underlie up to around 70% of the variability in fat mass observed in the population. Other than a very small number of individuals with rare recessive conditions such as those which disrupt leptin or its receptor, most individuals rendered susceptible to the modern "obesogenic environment" would have been rendered so through innumerable subtle alterations in an array of different genes, contributing to individual differences in energy absorption and dissipation. The ultimate goals of obesity genetics will be to unravel physiological pathways regulating energy balance (e.g., from examining the functions of non-candidate genes implicated in genome-wide association studies such as *FTO*), provide pharmacologic targets for drug development (recombinant leptin was the first specific treatment for a genetic obesity syndrome), and determine degrees of individual susceptibility to the obesogenic environment. The fact that all the known mutations discovered by genome-wide

Table 2.1 Other human pleiotropic obesity syndromes.

Syndrome	Additional clinical features	Locus
Albright hereditary osteodystrophy (AHO)/ McCune–Albright syndrome	Short stature, skeletal defects, and impaired olfaction. Also multiple hormone resistance when paternally transmitted. *GNAS1* gene mutation	20q13.3
Bardet–Biedl syndrome (BBS)	Mental retardation, dysmorphic extremities (syndactyly, brachydactyly, or polydactyly), retinal dystrophy or pigmentary retinopathy, hypogonadism or hypogenitalism (limited to male patients), and structural abnormalities of the kidney or functional renal impairment. The differential diagnosis includes Biemond syndrome II (iris coloboma, hypogenitalism, obesity, polydactyly, and mental retardation) and Alstrom syndrome (retinitis pigmentosa, obesity, diabetes mellitus, and deafness)	11q13
Ulnar–mammary syndrome	Ulnar defects, delayed puberty, and hypoplastic nipples	12q24.1
Alstrom syndrome	Retinal dystrophy, neurosensory deafness, and diabetes	2p13
Cohen syndrome	Prominent central incisors, ophthalmopathy, and microcephaly	8q22
Borjeson–Forssman–Lehmann syndrome	Mental retardation, hypogonadism, and large ears	Xq26
Fragile X syndrome	Moderate to severe mental retardation, macro-orchidism, large ears, prominent jaw, and high-pitched jocular speech associated with mutations in the *FMR1* gene. Expression is variable, with mental retardation being the most common feature. Behavioral characteristics include hyperkinesis, autistic-like behavior, and speech and language deficits	Xq27.3
MEHMO syndrome	Mental retardation, epilepsy, hypogonadism, and microcephaly	Xp22.13
Simpson–Golabi–Behmel, type 2	Craniofacial defects and skeletal and visceral abnormalities	Xp22
Wilson–Turner syndrome	Mental retardation, tapering fingers, and gynecomastia	Xp21.1

association studies to date, if all held by any one individual, would only add a few percentage points to their risk is perhaps disappointing, although in the future, perhaps by targeting phenotypes more aligned with genetic inheritance than the composite measure of BMI, some of the complexity may begin to unravel.

Pitfalls

- Consider genetic syndromes where there is a strong family history particularly of severe early-onset obesity or where there are other physical or developmental clues, for example, learning difficulties, small hands, hypogonadism, and very rapid or very impaired growth.
- Failing to explore a patient's perception of the origins of their obesity and what they are able to do to combat it—unexplored beliefs about genetic inevitability are unlikely to result in successful weight management.
- If you find it easier to adopt a non-judgmental approach to a known carrier of a genetic mutation, reflect on how many other individuals may carry other unknown or untested mutations, which together may contribute to the 40–70% heritability of obesity.
- Forty percent of the variance in resting metabolic rate, thermic effect of food, and energy cost of low- to moderate-intensity exercise may be explained by inherited characteristics.

Key web links

On-line Mendelian Inheritance in Man. http://www.ncbi.nlm.nih.gov/omim [accessed on December 29, 2012].

Centers for Disease Control and Prevention. http://www.cdc.gov/Features/Obesity/ [accessed on December 29, 2012].

Endotext Article, "The Genetics of Obesity in Humans," Stephen O'Rahilly and I. Sadaf Farooqi. http://www.endotext.org/obesity/obesity8/obesity8.htm [accessed on December 29, 2012].

Further reading

Aslan, I.R., Campos, G.M., Calton, M.A., *et al.* (2011) Weight loss after Roux-en-Y gastric bypass in obese patients heterozygous for MC4R mutations. *Obesity Surgery*, 21, 930–934.

Beales, P.L. (2010) Obesity in single gene disorders. *Progress in Molecular Biology and Translational Science*, 94, 125–157.

Blakemore, A.I., Froguel, P. (2010) Investigation of Mendelian forms of obesity holds out the prospect of personalized medicine. *Annals of the New York Academy of Sciences*, 1214, 180–189.

Bouchard, C. (2008) Gene-environment interactions in the etiology of obesity: Defining the fundamentals. *Obesity (Silver Spring)*, 16 (Suppl. 3), S5–S10.

Chambers, J.C., Elliott, P., Zabaneh, D. *et al.* (2008) Common genetic variation near MC4R is associated with waist circumference and insulin resistance. *Nature Genetics*, 40, 716–718.

Farooqi, I.S. (2008) Monogenic human obesity. *Frontiers Hormonal Research*, 36, 1–11.

Farooqi, I.S. (2011) Genetic, molecular and physiological insights into human obesity. *European Journal of Clinical Investigation*, 41, 451–455.

Frayling, T.M., Timpson, N.J., Weedon, M.N. *et al.* (2007) A common variant in the FTO gene is associated with body mass index and predisposes to childhood and adult obesity. *Science*, 316, 889–894.

Kousta, E., Hadjiathanasiou, C.G., Tolis, G. *et al.* (2009) Pleiotropic genetic syndromes with developmental abnormalities associated with obesity. *Journal of Pediatric Endocrinology & Metabolism*, 22, 581–592.

Levin, B.E. (2007) Why some of us get fat and what we can do about it. *Journal of Physiology*, 583(Pt 2), 425–430.

Mathes, W.F., Kelly, S.A., Pomp, D. (2011) Advances in comparative genetics: Influence of genetics on obesity. *British Journal of Nutrition*, 106 (Suppl. 1), S1–S10.

Paz-Filho, G., Wong, M.L., Licinio, J. (2011) Ten years of leptin replacement therapy. *Obesity Reviews*, 12, e315–e323.

Ramachandrappa, S., Farooqi, I.S. (2011) Genetic approaches to understanding human obesity. *Journal of Clinical Investigation* 121, 2080–2086.

Rankinen, T., Bouchard, C. (2008) Gene-physical activity interactions: Overview of human studies. *Obesity (Silver Spring)*, 16 (Suppl. 3), S47–S50.

Travers, M.E., McCarthy, M.I. (2011) Type 2 diabetes and obesity: Genomics and the clinic. *Human Genetics*, 130, 41–58.

CHAPTER 3

Adipocyte Biology

> **Key points**
> - White adipose tissue (WAT) is a regulated and co-ordinated endocrine organ displaying a multiplicity of, and regional variation in, function beyond its classical role in energy storage.
> - The expansion of WAT mass, the hallmark of obesity, has consequences on cardio-metabolic risk partly mediated by fatty acid uptake and release and also partly via local and systemic secretion of adipokines.
> - BAT has been identified in adult humans, is densely innervated by the SNS, and may play a significant role in adaptive thermogenesis.
> - Futile cycling of fatty acids within adipose tissue and uncoupled oxidative phosphory-lation are WAT-mediated mechanisms through which metabolic inefficiency may act to defend body weight.
> - Obesity is a pro-inflammatory state. This may be due to an adipose tissue depot outgrowing its blood supply causing tissue hypoxemia and the release of inflammatory cytokines from white adipocytes themselves or from reticulo-endothelial cells found within adipose tissue depots. Such inflammation is likely to contribute to endothelial dysfunction and to the vascular risk of obesity, as well as to erectile dysfunction (ED).

CASE STUDIES

Case study 1

ML, a 43-year-old journalist with a BMI of 32.5 kg/m², recently underwent a screening medical examination. She was told she had an elevated highly sensitive C-reactive protein (CRP). She had no signs of infection at the time and was told that this could indicate an increased risk of cardiovascular disease (CVD) even though her glucose tolerance test, blood pressure, and serum lipid profile had been optimized on appropriate treatment. She was advised by the screening nurse to consult you for further information.

Comment: You explain that obesity appears to lead to a chronic inflammatory state, reflected by highly sensitive CRP measurement, which may be linked to increased risk

Practical Manual of Clinical Obesity, First Edition. Robert Kushner, Victor Lawrence and Sudhesh Kumar.
© 2013 John Wiley & Sons, Ltd. Published 2013 by John Wiley & Sons, Ltd.

of CVD. This may be due in part to hypoxia of the expanded adipose tissue mass, which outstrips the ability of its blood supply to perfuse it. You explain that a single measurement of CRP in one particular individual may be elevated for a number of reasons and should be interpreted with caution. On the other hand, the result may serve as a useful reminder that, important though it is to optimize treatment of obesity-related risk factors, a residual risk will remain by virtue of the obesity itself and is likely to have an inflammatory basis.

Case study 2

DG, a 56-year-old smoker with a BMI of 31.9 kg/m², reports the development of ED over the past year, which has responded only partially to sildenafil. His primary physician has identified serum total testosterone levels right at the bottom of the reference range and is considering replacement. The patient was indignant when it was suggested by his primary physician that his problem may be related to his obesity and lifestyle, feeling that all health-care professionals tend to attribute every problem he ever has on his obesity and smoking.

Comment: You explain that ED is strongly associated with the metabolic syndrome; the more the features of this are present, the more likely ED is to be reported. You go on to explain that it is currently thought that pro-inflammatory cytokines released from an expanded fat mass in obesity (and from smoking) may cause endothelial dysfunction (directly affecting the vascular changes responsible for tumescence), reduce Leydig cell responsiveness to luteinizing hormone (LH) in the testis (reducing testosterone), and also reduce gonadotropin secretion (again, tending to reduce testosterone levels). There is increased conversion of testosterone by aromatase in adipose tissue into estrogen, which feeds back negatively on LH release, thereby inhibiting testosterone secretion. Furthermore, testosterone is bound to sex hormone–binding globulin (SHBG) which falls in obesity and insulin resistance, often reducing the measured levels of serum total testosterone. You explore anxieties he has about his general health, exclude depression, and explain that exercise may be beneficial. Following his new understanding of the significance of his symptom, you arrange to screen him for aspects of the metabolic syndrome (diabetes, hypertension, dyslipidemia, etc.) and discuss a realistic and achievable weight management and smoking cessation regime with his active engagement alongside the treatment options being explored by his primary care physician.

Introduction

WAT is more than a passive storage depot for fat: it is a regulated and co-ordinated endocrine organ with effects on energy intake, energy dissipation, and metabolic function. These effects have the potential to influence both the development and maintenance of obesity as well as cardiovascular and other complications of the obese state. BAT has distinct functions and may have more of a role in the adult human than has hitherto been thought.

Table 3.1 Non-classical functions of WAT.

WAT function	Examples
Function as an integrated organ	Contains different cell types with interdependent function. Regional heterogeneity of adipose tissue stores is well established, for example, the greater consequences of visceral versus subcutaneous adipose tissue accumulation in metabolic syndrome risk
Endocrine, paracrine, and autocrine functions	For example, leptin and TNF-α production, estrogen and cortisol metabolism, inhibition of lipolysis by free (non-esterified) fatty acid accumulation, and many others
Thermal insulation	Striking in some animals, for example, seals, and may be significant in some humans
Mechanical insulation	For example, of the eye within the orbits
Immune-, inflammation-, and fertility-related functions	Interaction with local lympho-reticular tissues, elaboration of pro-inflammatory cytokines, and permissive effect of leptin on gonadotropin secretion
TAG clearance from the blood stream	Lipodystrophic individuals are usually severely hyperlipidemic
Storage of other compounds including drugs	Amiodarone, mitotane, and so on

Expansion of WAT is the hallmark of obesity. The origins of obesity essentially stem from the triad of
1 appetite (energy intake)
2 adaptive components of energy expenditure
3 adipocyte biology
In lean subjects, WAT typically contributes less than 25% of body mass. This proportion ranges right across the lipodystrophic to adiposity spectrum, demonstrating the huge variability of the size of WAT stores. Triacylglycerol (TAG) is more energy dense than protein or carbohydrate, and no additional water is needed; hence, it is the preferred form of energy storage within the body, with liver glycogen stores becoming deplete within hours of entering the fasting (post-absorptive) state. In addition to its role in fat (TAG) storage, it has become clear that WAT has many other roles, including those listed in Table 3.1.

TAG storage and release

Adipose tissue removes TAG from the circulation. TAG may be released from circulating lipoproteins via the action of the enzyme lipoprotein

Table 3.2 Examples of adipokines released from WAT and their principal effect(s).

Adipokine	Principal effect(s)
Leptin	Energy balance, appetite and obesity, and immune and reproductive functions
Angiotensin	Blood pressure regulation—potential role in obesity-related hypertension
PAI-1	Coagulation, hypercoagulability, and inflammation
IL-1β	Inflammation and immunity
TNF-α	Inflammation and immunity
VEGF	Angiogenesis
IL-6	Insulin sensitivity
Adiponectin	Insulin sensitivity

lipase (LPL) or may be synthesized from free fatty acids (FFAs) or from glucose or other substrates in a high-carbohydrate/low-fat diet. Release of FFA from stored TAG in adipose tissue is largely (but not completely) dependent on the action of hormone-sensitive lipase (HSL), which is regulated most immediately by insulin and the SNS. Some of the released FFAs are re-esterified in what amounts to a futile cycle, dissipating energy. Exercise and activation of the SNS may have a role in the regulation of such futile cycles via the local accumulation of FFA in conditions of low adipose tissue blood flow and their subsequent re-uptake and re-esterification. To what extent such futile cycling contributes to the overall energy balance homeostasis of a given individual is at present uncertain.

Secretory function of WAT

Fatty acids are released from stored lipids in WAT. Cholesterol and prostaglandins are synthesized, and retinol and other compounds including drugs and toxins (e.g., organophosphates) are stored and may later be released. WAT has a function in the conversion of inactive 11-ketosteroids to active glucocorticoids via 11-β hydroxysteroid dehydrogenase type I. This may be excessive in obesity, and the term "Cushing disease of the omentum" has been advanced to describe this concept.

Leptin, TNF-α, adipsin, and over 60 other adipokines are released from WAT. Some of these and their principal effects are listed in Table 3.2.

These effects range from those which may have relevance to the achievement and maintenance of the obese state to those which may increase the metabolic and vascular consequences of obesity. Perhaps the most important are effects that concern energy balance and insulin sensitivity.

Adipokine effects on energy balance

Leptin signals the size of the fat stores and interacts with orexigenic (appetite-stimulating) pathways, for example, NPY and AgRP, and anorexigenic (appetite-inhibiting) pathways, for example, POMC and CART. Overall, energy intake and storage is increased in response to low leptin levels. Leptin also has effects mediated in part through the SNS. High levels may increase energy expenditure through adaptive thermogenesis (Chapter 1). Leptin levels are generally proportional to the size of the fat mass in obesity and, in most cases, well beyond the sloped part of the dose–response curve. Thus, for most obese individuals, further leptin secretion produces little or no further effect on increasing energy intake and reducing energy dissipation. Whether a degree of leptin resistance (e.g., poor penetration into the CNS) or relative leptin deficiency (lower levels than expected for adipose tissue mass) may contribute in some minor way to obesity in some subjects remains uncertain, but, at present, leptin appears to have little potential for use as an anti-obesity agent save for the very rare cases reported in the world literature of congenital absolute leptin deficiency.

Adiponectin levels fall in obesity. High levels stimulate energy expenditure and increase the corticotropin-releasing hormone (CRH). Interleukin-6 (IL-6) is thought to have a role in insulin resistance, and its levels increase in parallel with the fat mass.

Adipokine effects on insulin sensitivity

Both too much and too little WAT are associated with insulin resistance. The administration of either leptin or adiponectin to lipodystrophic animals is able to increase insulin sensitivity. Other adipokines including visfatin, resistin, and retinol-binding protein (RBP-4) may also mediate the relationship between adiposity and insulin resistance.

Adipokine effects on inflammation

Chronic low-grade inflammation is present in obesity. This is reflected in measures of inflammation, including highly sensitive CRP and PAI-1. Increased spillover of these pro-inflammatory cytokines from adipose tissue into the circulation has been shown experimentally in human obesity. T2DM and CVD have long been recognized as being pro-inflammatory states, and some obesity-related cancers including breast cancer may have inflammatory components. Interleukins 1β, 6, 8, 10, and 18 as well as MCP-1, MIF, TGF-β, TNF-α, PAI-1, haptoglobin, serum amyloid A, NFG, and adiponectin have all been hypothesized to link obesity with these inflammatory complications. The levels of all of these markers increase with increasing fat mass, with the exception of adiponectin. Many of these adipokines may be released from within WAT but by infiltrating macrophages and other reticulo-endothelial cells found within WAT rather than directly from white adipocytes themselves. The precise reason for the increased inflammation found as WAT mass expands is not known, but possible explanations include

a a response to endoplasmic reticulum stress

b a response to oxidative stress

c a response to hypoxia

Hypoxia might underlie all of these putative mechanisms, and it has been suggested that hypoxia within adipose tissue may arise due to a mismatch between the expanded fat depot and its blood supply. If this is indeed the case, adipocytes and other cells distant from the vasculature would experience hypoxemic conditions, which would give rise to a cellular response, including stimulation of inflammation and angiogenesis. Emerging data do suggest that WAT is indeed hypoxic in obesity, stimulating excessive production of VEGF, HIF-1, PAI-1, and other pro-inflammatory mediators.

Brown adipose tissue (BAT)

Brown adipose tissue (BAT) is present only in mammals. It differs from WAT in both form and function, as described in Table 3.3.

In the past, it was thought that this fat type was present only in human infants. More recent FDG-PET scanning data have confirmed however that

Table 3.3 Comparison of BAT and WAT.

BAT	WAT
Only present in mammals	Not restricted to mammals
Small amounts in humans after infancy (although more than previously thought)	Much more variable amounts depending on energy stores
Multiple droplets per adipocyte	Single large lipid droplet per cell
Fat content 20–40% of cell volume	Fat content 80% of cell volume
Luxuriant vascularization	Good vascularization except, perhaps, when grossly expanded
Extensive SNS innervation and β3-adrenoceptor expression	Direct SNS innervation sparse if at all present. Little β3-adrenoceptor expression in humans
Many mitochondria	Few mitochondria
Abundant uncoupling protein (UCP-1) expression	No UCP-1 expression
Prominent role in heat generation	No direct role in heat generation (some role in insulation)

BAT is indeed present in adult humans (especially in the inter-scapular adipose tissue depot) and is found in large amounts in patients with pheo-chromocytoma. This suggests that

a brown fat is present in adults

b brown fat quantity may be linked to the activity of the SNS and is inducible

c the ability to form brown fat is not lost in adulthood, merely suppressed

BAT appears to have a primary role in heat generation via uncoupling of oxidative phosphorylation, that is, the leaching of chemical and electrical energy as heat as a form of "adaptive" metabolic inefficiency. This would seem potentially useful in counteracting obesity, although to what extent this actually happens in humans is presently unclear.

Conclusion

Adipocytes are endocrine and secretory cells. WAT is the largest organ in the obese individual. Inflammation may be a characteristic of an expanded fat mass, and the mechanism may be cellular stress due to hypoxia aris-ing from increasing distance of some cells from their nearest blood supply. BAT is a distinct tissue whose role in adult obesity is being reassessed in the light of the fact that it is a potential source of energy dissipation through heat, is present in the adult human, and may be inducible by SNS activation.

Pitfalls

- Beta-blockers may inhibit some beneficial effects of the SNS and lead to weight gain (up to 4 kg or 9 lb in some studies)—consider alternative treatments where appropriate.
- Be sure to emphasize physiological actions, for example, of adipokines rather than "moralistic" explanations when discussing the causes and consequences of a patient's obesity.
- ED may indicate a pro-inflammatory state and indicate the presence of the metabolic syndrome and increased overall cardiovascular risk.
- Be alert to the possibility of low testosterone levels in obesity.
- Be mindful of the potential for the accumulation of lipid-soluble drugs, for example, amiodarone or mitotane, and other pharmacokinetic effects of excess adipose tissue accumulation in obese individuals.
- Advise obese patients to avoid other precipitants of inflammation, for example, smoking.
- BAT may be inducible by the action of the SNS and can dissipate energy in the form of heat. Consider the possible benefits of, for example, turning down the central heating, which may induce an increase in this fat type.

Key web links

NIDDK. http://www2.niddk.nih.gov/Research/ScientificAreas/Diabetes/MetabolismAnd IntegrativePhysiology/ADIP.htm [accessed on December 29, 2012].

Further reading

Bartness, T.J. & Song, C.K. (2007) Thematic review series: Adipocyte biology. Sympathetic and sensory innervation of white adipose tissue. *Journal of Lipid Research*, 48, 1655–1672.

Bartness, T.J., Vaughan, C.H. & Song, C.K. (2010) Sympathetic and sensory innervation of brown adipose tissue. *International Journal of Obesity (London)*, 34 (Suppl. 1), S36–S42.

Eizirik, D.L., Cardozo, A.K. & Cnop, M. (2008) The role for endoplasmic reticulum stress in diabetes mellitus. *Endocrine Reviews*, 29, 42–61.

Gleeson, M., Bishop, N.C., Stensel, D.J., Lindley, M.R., Mastana, S.S. & Nimmo, M.A. (2011) The anti-inflammatory effects of exercise: Mechanisms and implications for the prevention and treatment of disease. *Nature Reviews Immunology*, 11, 607–615.

Gregor, M.F. & Hotamisligil, G.S. (2011) Inflammatory mechanisms in obesity. *Annual Review of Immunology*, 29, 415–445.

Lumeng, C.N. & Saltiel, A.R. (2011) Inflammatory links between obesity and metabolic disease. *Journal of Clinical Investigation*, 121, 2111–2117.

Maury, E. & Brichard, S.M. (2010) Adipokine dysregulation, adipose tissue inflammation and metabolic syndrome. *Molecular and Cellular Endocrinology*, 314, 1–16.

Morton, N.M. & Seckl, J.R. (2008) 11beta-hydroxysteroid dehydrogenase type 1 and obesity. *Frontiers of Hormone Research*, 36, 146–164.

Nedergaard, J., Bengtsson, T. & Cannon, B. (2010) Three years with adult human brown adipose tissue. *Annals of New York Academy of Sciences*, 1212, E20–E36.

Rasouli, N. & Kern, P.A. (2008) Adipocytokines and the metabolic complications of obesity. *Journal of Clinical Endocrinology and Metabolism*, 93 (Suppl. 1), S64–S73.

Rosen, E.D. & Spiegelman, B.M. (2006) Adipocytes as regulators of energy balance and glucose homeostasis. *Nature*, 444, 847–853.

Tamler, R. & Deveney, T. (2010) Hypogonadism, erectile dysfunction, and type 2 diabetes mellitus: What the clinician needs to know. *Postgraduate Medicine*, 122, 165–175.

Wood, I.S., de Heredia, F.P., Wang, B. & Trayhurn, P. (2009) Cellular hypoxia and adipose tissue dysfunction in obesity. *Proceedings of the Nutrition Society*, 68, 370–377. Review.

CHAPTER 4

Fetal and Infant Origins of Obesity

Key points

It is now clear that factors operating in early pregnancy or even before may influence later risk of obesity. Some of these factors may tend to amplify the obesity epidemic ("obesity begets obesity"), and some but not all are potentially modifiable. Despite inherent study limitations and problems in ascertaining accurate length/height in early childhood, a consensus view from the available data at the present time would be as follows:

- Maternal weight loss during pregnancy and reduced fetal birth weight are likely to be harmful.
- Smoking cessation is highly desirable (before, during, and after pregnancy).
- Gestational diabetes mellitus (GDM) may be prevented in some cases by exercise before or during pregnancy and by entering pregnancy at an ideal body weight. It is not yet clear whether treatment of GDM itself reduces the increased fetal risk of later obesity, but it clearly improves fetal outcome.
- Breastfeeding has numerous well-established benefits and is clearly the preferred infant nutrition where possible. Some data suggest that prolonged breastfeeding may produce an increasing cumulative risk reduction for later obesity in the infant, although not all studies have shown this effect. Certainly, breastfeeding does not increase the risk of infant obesity, and it may possibly reduce it.
- Rapid weight gain in infancy has been linked to a possible increase in the later risk of obesity, although there are insufficient data at the present time for general recommendations and some concerns that misguided advice to slow down catch-up weight gain may, in some circumstances, for example, pre-term infants, risk impairing neuro-cognitive outcomes in these infants.

CASE STUDIES

Case study 1

SB, a 29-year-old woman with a BMI of 31 kg/m², consults you after being recently diagnosed with GDM. She asks whether this could have an effect on her baby's risk of obesity or diabetes.

Practical Manual of Clinical Obesity, First Edition. Robert Kushner, Victor Lawrence and Sudhesh Kumar.
© 2013 John Wiley & Sons, Ltd. Published 2013 by John Wiley & Sons, Ltd.

Comment: You enquire about other risk factors, specifically her family history of both conditions, and acknowledge that there is a slightly increased risk by virtue of the diagnosis. However, any additional risk (beyond that which would already have been genetically determined) would be outweighed in many ways by its early identification with the potential to prevent or counteract it in both mother and child both during and after pregnancy. The benefits of good control of gestational diabetes are well established, and this would involve limiting weight gain during pregnancy; taking part in exercise appropriate for the stage of pregnancy, for example, walking; and using diet and medication (e.g., insulin, metformin where appropriate) to optimize blood glucose levels and prevent fetal macrosomia. Close monitoring of fetal growth and development and optimal timing of delivery would also be undertaken. Breastfeeding is beneficial for many reasons including weight control in both mother and infant, as is a healthy active lifestyle, starting perhaps with daily walks as soon as possible after delivery.

Case study 2

CM, a 24-year-old woman with a strong family history of obesity and diabetes, has recently had her first pregnancy confirmed with an estimated gestation of 7 weeks. Her BMI is 27.3 kg/m². She asks if there is anything she can do during pregnancy and early infancy to reduce her child's risk of becoming obese and/or developing diabetes later in life.

Comment: You take a full history and discover that she is a smoker. You explain that smoking may impair blood flow to the baby in the womb and may lead to low birth weight, which, among other known risks, may favor the expression of a "thrifty phenotype" predisposed to efficient accumulation of energy and therefore obesity. You advise her that limiting weight gain during pregnancy, breastfeeding, eating a healthy diet, and taking regular exercise may have beneficial effects on setting the baby's metabolism for the future as may provision of sufficient time for sleep. You discuss ways of encouraging healthy activity in the child and limiting the intake of "empty calories," such as those found in calorie-rich drinks.

Introduction

Although the diagnosis and management of obesity in childhood is outside the remit of this discussion, it is increasingly clear that events before conception, during pregnancy, and in very early infant life have lasting effects on body composition. It is therefore important to have some understanding of the practical and methodological issues inherent in assessing and defining obesity in early childhood and in linking such anthropomorphic data to events later on in life. Genetic factors are discussed elsewhere; the focus of the present chapter is on the pre-natal, intra-uterine, infant, and childhood environmental determinants of obesity. The major current conceptual frameworks of "life course" and "developmental origins" are discussed.

Measurement

As with adults, BMI is a convenient measure of obesity in children but has drawbacks of being poorly applicable to children under the age of 2, largely due to difficulties inherent in accurate length/height measurement in young children (with a tendency to over-estimate) and in poor correlations with adiposity particularly at the lower percentiles of BMI. Under the age of 2 years, Centre for Disease Control (CDC) or World Health Organization (WHO) weight-for-length charts are commonly used, with overweight and obesity being defined in those exceeding the 85th and 95th percentiles, respectively.

In research practice, measures of body composition may be preferable. Dual-energy X-ray absorptiometry (DEXA) and PEA POD (infant-sized air-displacement plethysmograph) techniques may be used, although DEXA is constrained by the need to administer a small dose of radiation. Skinfold thickness measurement is safe and convenient and, in well-trained hands, gives a reasonable estimate of body fat content. Bioimpedance measurements are not accurate in very young children.

Conceptual framework of early origins of obesity

The two most prevalent conceptual frameworks linking environmental events early in life to later obesity and its complications are the so-called "Life Course" and developmental origins theories, which are introduced as follows.

Life course approach to chronic diseases

This theory holds that external (environmental) factors act in the pre-conceptual, pre-natal, infant, and childhood phases of development. These factors interact and have different importance at different stages of development. "Programming" is said to exist when a particular factor exerts its influence at a critical or sensitive developmental stage and leads to lasting or permanent consequences, for example, maternal GDM. "Risk" accrues when a particular factor is present over a longer time frame, for example, chronic exposure to elevated serum lipid concentrations risks later predisposition to atherosclerosis.

Developmental origins of health and disease (DOHaD)

The DOHaD theory focuses on the pre-natal period and early infancy and is concerned with exposures that are complete by the first years of life. Later factors only modify the trajectories set by the earlier events. An example of this conceptualization is the increased cardiovascular risk of low-birth-weight infants, often referred to as the "thrifty phenotype hypothesis."

Modifiable developmental disease determinants

Experimental data relating early events to the later development of disease (e.g., by uterine artery ligation to cause fetal malnutrition) are difficult to obtain in humans for obvious reasons, and prospective cohort data may take many years to obtain even if the right questions were asked and the correct data stored. Observational data suffer from confoundment and may be difficult to interpret. Nevertheless, despite all these limitations, it is becoming increasingly possible to identify a number of modifiable developmental disease determinants and advise patients and populations accordingly. These have been summarized in a recent workshop report—"Influence of Pregnancy Weight on Maternal and Child Health: Workshop Report"—from the Institute of Medicine (IOM) and National Research Council (see Key web links), and some of these are now discussed.

Pre-natal modifiable determinants

Modifiable factors acting *in utero* include the following:

1 High maternal pre-pregnancy BMI and gestational weight gain are both associated with childhood overweight. Recommendations for maternal gestational weight gain dependent on pre-pregnancy BMI have recently been produced by the IOM (see Table 4.1 and Key web links).

2 Fetal nutrition (dependent on maternal nutrition, uterine blood flow, and other factors).

3 Maternal smoking (50% increased adjusted odds ratio for obesity in affected offspring).

4 GDM (a possible factor in the amplification of the obesity epidemic: maternal obesity leading to fetal macrosomia and late effects including increased fetal risk of obesity and diabetes mellitus). Gestational diabetes risk is known to be reduced with appropriate exercise before and during early pregnancy and with limitation of pregnancy-associated weight gain. The adverse fetal effects of maternal GDM are known to be reduced by diagnosis and appropriate management of the condition. The risk of the mother going on to develop T2DM may be reduced by appropriate dietary counseling and

Table 4.1 Recommendations for maternal gestational weight gain dependent on pre-pregnancy BMI as recommended by the IOM

Pre-pregnancy weight class	Recommended weight gain (lb/kg)
Normal (BMI 18.5–24.9 kg/m²)	25–35 lb (11.4–15.9 kg)
Overweight (BMI 25–29.9 kg/m²)	15–25 lb (6.8–11.4 kg)
Obese (BMI > 30 kg/m²)	11–20 lb (5–9.1 kg)

exercise programs, and pharmacotherapy, for example, with metformin, may be considered alongside these interventions. Testing for the condition 6 weeks after delivery and annually thereafter for life is generally advised.

Post-natal modifiable determinants

1 *Infant growth (specifically weight gain in excess of linear growth).* Increased obesity risk has been shown in one study even when excessive growth occurred in just the first week of life in formula-fed infants, including those showing "catch-up growth." However, it is important to add that other studies have been conflicting in this regard and on present evidence, the well-established benefits, for example, in neuro-cognitive outcomes of pre-term infants who achieve rapid catch-up growth should not be denied them on the basis of a putative risk of later obesity.

2 *Infant nutrition.* Breastfeeding has been shown in one study to reduce obesity by 4% for each month of breastfeeding with a total possible risk reduction of 13–22%. However, this finding appears limited to a White US population, and other studies have shown conflicting results. Nevertheless, it appears reasonable on the basis of current data to conclude that breastfeeding does not increase the risk of later developing obesity and may perhaps reduce it. There is some evidence that failure to initiate or to sustain breastfeeding may be associated with raised pre-pregnancy BMI and excessive gestational weight gain, although whether this association is causal is unclear.

3 *Sleep duration.* In adults, reduced sleep correlates with increased obesity risk. In infants, sleeping for less than 12 h a day doubles the obesity risk of the child at 3 years.

Combination of pre- and post-natal factors

Combinations of
1 smoking
2 greater maternal weight increase during pregnancy
3 breastfeeding duration, and
4 infant sleep
have been proven in one study to be a powerful predictor of later obesity, conferring an absolute risk of 6% with optimal levels of all factors and 29% with adverse levels of all risks, with a continuum of risk in between these two extremes, as depicted in Figure 4.1.

Summary

Events taking place during pregnancy and in early childhood may act either at a critical point in development or over a period of time to change

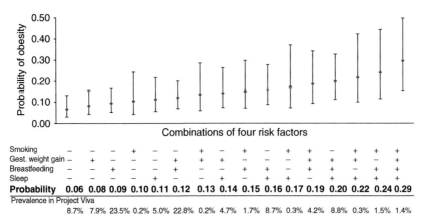

Smoking	–	–	–	+	–	–	+	–	+	–	+	+	–	+	+	+
Gest. weight gain	–	+	–	–	–	+	+	+	–	–	–	+	+	+	–	+
Breastfeeding	–	–	+	+	–	+	–	–	+	+	–	+	+	–	+	+
Sleep	–	–	–	–	+	–	–	+	–	+	+	–	+	+	+	+
Probability	**0.06**	**0.08**	**0.09**	**0.10**	**0.11**	**0.12**	**0.13**	**0.14**	**0.15**	**0.16**	**0.17**	**0.19**	**0.20**	**0.22**	**0.24**	**0.29**
Prevalence in Project Viva	8.7%	7.9%	23.5%	0.2%	5.0%	22.8%	0.2%	4.7%	1.7%	8.7%	0.3%	4.2%	8.8%	0.3%	1.5%	1.4%

Figure 4.1 Predicted probability of obesity (BMI greater than 95th percentile) at 3 years of age for 16 combinations of 4 modifiable risk factors during pregnancy and infancy. Bars show 95% confidence limits. Also shown is prevalence for each depicted combination of factors among 1110 mother–child pairs participating in Project Viva. Probabilities are adjusted for maternal education and BMI, household income, and child race/ethnicity. Reproduced from Kopelman *et al.* (eds) (2010) *Clinical Obesity in Adults and Children*, 3rd edn, Blackwell Publishing, Oxford, with permission from Blackwell Publishing.

susceptibility to later obesity and its associated metabolic disorders. Some of these influences (e.g., maternal body weight, smoking, infant feeding, diagnosis and management of GDM) are modifiable and some (e.g., some gene–environment interactions) may not be. Increased understanding of the developmental origins of disease will pave the way for better individual- and population-based strategies for harm reduction and has the potential to break the cycle through which the consequences of obesity may be passed on to future generations.

Pitfalls

- Missing the opportunity to plan for pregnancy in women who are overweight or, even more importantly, have diabetes. In obese women, such planning would include institution of diet and exercise modification prior to pregnancy, discussion of the potential risks to both mother and child, and, to the extent it is achievable, attainment of an ideal or at least improved body weight. In women with diabetes, optimization of glycemic control, control of co-morbidities (e.g., retinopathy, renal dysfunction), the use of folic acid, and avoidance of drugs that may affect pregnancy are also crucially important.
- Failing to recognize the greatly increased risk of developing T2DM in women who have had gestational diabetes.
- Failing to consider the importance of the (potentially modifiable) intra-uterine environment in the pathogenesis of obesity.

Key web links

Institute of Medicine Report. http://www.iom.edu/Reports/2007/Influence-of-Pregnancy-Weight-on-Maternal-and-Child-Health--A-Workshop-Report.aspx [accessed on December 29, 2012].

Institute of Medicine Report. http://www.iom.edu/Reports/2009/Weight-Gain-During-Pregnancy-Reexamining-the-Guidelines.aspx [accessed on December 29, 2012].

National Institute for Health and Clinical Excellence. Guideline for the management of diabetes in pregnancy from preconception to the postnatal period. http://www.nice.org.uk/CG063fullguideline [accessed on December 29, 2012].

Centre for Maternal and Child Enquiries and the Royal College of Obstetricians and Gynaecologists Guideline 'Management of Women with Obesity in Pregnancy'. http://www.rcog.org.uk/files/rcog-corp/CMACERCOGJointGuidelineManagementWomen ObesityPregnancya.pdf [accessed on December 29, 2012].

Further reading

Calkins, K. & Devaskar, S.U. (2011) Fetal origins of adult disease. *Current Problems in Pediatric and Adolescent Health Care*, 41, 158–176.

McMillen, I.C., Rattanatray, L., Duffield, J.A. *et al.* (2009) The early origins of later obesity: Pathways and mechanisms. *Advances in Experimental Medicine and Biology*, 646, 71–81.

Muhlhausler, B.S. & Ong, Z.Y. (2011) The fetal origins of obesity: Early origins of altered food intake. *Endocrine, Metabolic & Immune Disorders Drug Targets*, 11, 189–197.

Ong, K.K. (2010) Early determinants of obesity. *Endocrine Development*, 19, 53–61.

Stocker, C.J., Arch, J.R. & Cawthorne, M.A. (2005) Fetal origins of insulin resistance and obesity. *Proceedings of the Nutrition Society*, 64, 143–151.

Wax, J.R. (2009) Risks and management of obesity in pregnancy: Current controversies. *Current Opinion in Obstetrics & Gynecology*, 21, 117–123.

CHAPTER 5

Metabolic Fuels and Obesity

Key points
- Following a mixed meal, the rate of appearance of both glucose and triglyceride into the circulation would be expected to increase some 10-fold were it not for rapid transition between the fasting and post-prandial states.
- Insulin acts as the main switch between these states.
- The tissues most involved in this transition and in the consequent nutrient partitioning (storage, release, and selection of metabolic fuels under differing metabolic circumstances) are
  - liver (glucose storage as glycogen, glucose production from gluconeogenetic precursors, lipoprotein production)
  - muscle (glucose uptake, glucose and fatty acid oxidation during exercise)
  - WAT (NEFA storage after eating and release during fasting or exercise)
- Transition between fasting and post-absorptive states may be delayed or incomplete in obesity (metabolic inflexibility). This may be a manifestation of insulin resistance.
- Overabundance of fat within skeletal muscle as intra-myocellular lipid is strongly correlated with impaired glucose disposal after a meal. Similarly, overabundance of fat within the liver is associated with impaired suppression of hepatic glucose output (HGO) in the fasting state. Both of these manifestations of "lipotoxicity" are hallmarks of the fasting and post-prandial hyperglycemia encountered in T2DM. Proposed mechanisms include adipokine effects, the Randle hypothesis (competition between glucose and lipid metabolism depending on substrate availability at the level of the Krebs cycle), and complex signal transduction interactions of lipid metabolites leading to insulin resistance.
- Metabolic fuel selection may vary as a result of diet, obesity, and training, tending to favor carbohydrate rather than fat metabolism in the obese and unfit individual.
- Inefficiency in lipolysis and fatty acid re-esterification (futile cycling) has been linked to SNS activity and may be a component of the metabolic inefficiency that leads to increased thermogenesis following experimental weight gain.
- It is important to appreciate the difference between *whole-body* nutrient fluxes and fluxes *per kilogram* of the tissue under study. Glucose disposal *per kilogram lean tissue* and lipolysis *per kilogram fat mass* are typically both reduced in obesity (largely as a consequence of insulin resistance), whereas *whole-body* glucose disposal and lipolysis are often increased due to the expansion of both lean and adipose tissues encountered in obesity.

Practical Manual of Clinical Obesity, First Edition. Robert Kushner, Victor Lawrence and Sudhesh Kumar.
© 2013 John Wiley & Sons, Ltd. Published 2013 by John Wiley & Sons, Ltd.

CASE STUDIES

Case study 1

Your patient, JS, is a 32-year-old obese man with a BMI of 33 kg/m². He has undertaken a program of diet and exercise following your last consultation and has joined a gym on your advice. He mentions to you that he has heard people at the gym talking about how "muscles can be made to burn more fat" through physical training and finds this concept potentially rather motivating. He asks whether this has a basis in science or whether it is just "gym talk."

Comment: You agree with him. The hallmark of the fit and insulin-sensitive individual is early use of lipid rather than glucose oxidation during exercise and of increased clearance of triglyceride from plasma by the exercising muscle, which contributes to an improved plasma lipid profile and in all likelihood to the improvement in insulin sensitivity seen with exercise. In addition, resting metabolic rate is increased for some time after exercise, giving rise to the motivating concept of continuing to "burn off calories" later on while sleeping, and, of course, there are the benefits in terms of overall energy expenditure and reduced cardiovascular risk that come from exercise. You caution him that exercise alone is rarely successful on its own as a form of weight management but that, combined with suitable dietary restriction, the changes he has made will be hugely beneficial in combating both his obesity and also its complications.

Case study 2

Another patient, KM is an obese 66-year-old retired teacher with a family history of T2DM and a BMI of 37 kg/m². You recently arranged a glucose tolerance test for him on the basis of an impaired fasting glucose result and have explained to him that he has "impaired fasting glucose" and "impaired glucose tolerance." You explain that his obesity on the background of a genetic predisposition has led him to develop insulin resistance and "pre-diabetes." He asks what exactly insulin does and what the consequences of his own abnormalities on insulin action might be. He feels that the explanation offered by another health professional that it "unlocks the door to cells so that glucose can enter" is insufficiently enlightening.

Comment: You explain that insulin acts as the major switch between the fasting and the fed states. In the fasting state, adipose tissue releases FFAs for oxidation or incorporation by the liver into lipoproteins. The liver produces glucose from other substrates in the process of gluconeogenesis and releases glucose from glycogen stores by glycogenolysis. Once calories are ingested, insulin is released, which increases glucose uptake predominantly into muscles by stimulation of a transporter protein, glucose transporter 4 (GLUT-4), which helps glucose cross the cell membranes. Glucose production and release by the liver is rapidly and almost completely suppressed as is the release of fatty acids by adipose tissue, which switches to lipid uptake and storage. The net effect of these changes in normal individuals is to "buffer" the rise in concentrations of both glucose and lipids in the bloodstream after a meal. In individuals with central obesity, excessive release of fatty acids may induce insulin resistance in the liver and interfere with insulin secretion from pancreatic beta cells. Hepatic production of glucose from stored glycogen (glycogenolysis) and *de novo* (gluconeogenesis) is increased, thus contributing to the fasting hyperglycemia that has been demonstrated by the tests that he has had. Insulin resistance in other tissues (predominantly muscle and adipose tissue) together with abnormal insulin secretion results in both glucose and lipid levels being higher for longer after eating as the transition between the fasting and post-prandial states becomes delayed and incomplete. This contributes to impaired glucose disposal after a glucose load and, thus, to impaired glucose tolerance that has been demonstrated in his tests. You explain that a combination of regular exercise and weight control with a mildly hypocaloric but balanced and healthy diet, avoiding excessive dietary fat intake, can counteract many of these changes and has been shown to be able to delay and most likely prevent the development of T2DM in many individuals with "pre-diabetes."

Introduction

Metabolism and fuel selection vary between tissues and in the same tissue under differing metabolic conditions. Changes in obesity may be seen either as adaptive or maladaptive depending on circumstances. T2DM has been postulated to be a defense against obesity (e.g., by limiting cellular glucose uptake and spilling excess calories into the urine) but is clearly maladaptive overall.

The focus of this chapter is to discuss the normal metabolic fuel selections of key tissues and to examine their transition between fasting (post-absorptive) and fed (post-prandial) states and their response to exercise at different intensities and durations in trained and sedentary individuals.

Physiological conditions in weight-stable individuals

The principal metabolic states that humans transition between in day-to-day life are

1 the fasting (post-absorptive) state
2 the fed (post-prandial) state
3 exercise

Transitions between these states occur over minutes (e.g., eating/starting exercise) or may be more gradual (e.g., returning to the post-absorptive state some hours after eating). A large proportion of a 24-h period is spent in this transition, and it is increasingly recognized that failure to transition normally may be a hallmark of obesity/insulin resistance.

Skeletal muscle and WAT are distributed throughout the body in depots that vary metabolically or histologically. Muscles vary in oxidative capacity, histology, glycogen stores, and TAG stores, and there are well-described differences, for example, in the higher metabolic risk conferred by a relative accumulation of visceral (central) upper body fat as opposed to gluteo-femoral or lower body subcutaneous fat, particularly as regards insulin resistance.

Fasting (post-absorptive) conditions

Fasting is for most people the predominant state occurring for approximately 8–12 h/day. During fasting, lipid oxidation becomes increasingly predominant as a source of energy with increasing duration of fasting as limited carbohydrate stores become depleted.

Muscle post-absorptive metabolism

Muscle accounts for approximately 40% of body weight in a typical or "reference" man and a little less (30%) in "reference woman." It may approach 65% in a trained athlete but tends to decrease as a proportion of total body mass with advancing age. Skeletal muscle is a major carbohydrate reservoir. The liver contains around 100 g stored as glycogen, but muscle contains some 400 g. However, the main fuel in muscle after an overnight fast is lipid.

Skeletal muscle is an important site for lipid clearance at rest and also during exercise. In obesity, muscle TAG stores increase. Some is stored in adipocytes within a muscle, some in muscle cells themselves (as intra-myocellular lipid), and there is a possibility of autocrine or paracrine interaction between muscle and adipose tissue at this level, which may have relevance to the development of muscle insulin resistance.

The Randle hypothesis was long ago advanced as a link between carbohydrate and fat metabolism. In its original version, competition between products of lipid metabolism (e.g., acetyl CoA, citrate) and glucose was thought to favor fat metabolism in conditions of abundant NEFA supply such as obesity, leading to impaired glucose disposal. More recent conceptualizations center more on the signal transduction effects of derivatives of fat metabolism, such as long-chain acyl CoA, diacylglycerol, and ceramides. Whatever the precise pathophysiological basis, it is widely accepted that overabundance of "ectopic" fat within skeletal muscle (e.g., as intra-myocellular lipid) is strongly associated with impaired glucose uptake and oxidation by insulin-dependent and non-insulin-dependent mechanisms.

Adipose tissue post-absorptive metabolism

"Reference man" has a body composition comprising some 20% body fat (30% in "reference woman"), although this may be as little as 9–12% in trained athletes. The accrual of additional fat is the most obvious change in obesity, although the concomitant expansion of lean body tissues in obesity is important, as is their loss during caloric restriction.

A consistent characteristic of the expanded adipose tissue mass in obesity is its relative metabolic inertness *per kilogram* compared to in the non-obese state, although the opposite effect may be seen when considering whole-body fluxes due to the absolute increase in the total body fat content. Visceral adipose tissue is relatively less inert in terms of net lipolysis in obesity, and the consequent delivery of NEFA to the liver in high concentrations via the portal vein is thought to be a potential link between central adiposity and insulin resistance, particularly the ability of insulin fully and promptly to suppress HGO.

Adipose tissue plays a small role in glucose disposal (approximately 5%), and the release of FFAs is its main metabolic role in the fasting state. This switches very rapidly from high release to close to 0 in lean subjects in the post-prandial state predominantly as a result of HSL inhibition by insulin.

Adipose tissue regulates fasting plasma TAG concentrations in two ways:

a Its rate of release of FFAs, particularly via the portal vein, regulates hepatic triglyceride secretion in very-low-density lipoprotein (VLDL) particles.

b Its extraction of plasma triglyceride (via the rate-limiting enzyme LPL) regulates plasma triglyceride levels.

Adipose tissue also affects energy metabolism via the secretion of peptides and adipokines, for example, leptin, which act locally or as hormones signaling to the brain, muscle, and other tissues.

Brown adipose tissue (BAT) makes a small contribution to body lipid fluxes, but its role in energy homeostasis is potentially important. It is densely innervated by the SNS and a source of thermogenesis via uncoupling of oxidative phosphorylation.

Liver post-absorptive metabolism

The liver increases glucose production from gluconeogenetic precursors (lactate, glycerol, and amino acids) in obesity. Increased HGO may lead to fasting hyperglycemia, a major contributor to the pathophysiology of T2DM. Increased NEFA delivery to the liver may cause non-alcoholic fatty liver disease (NAFLD), insulin resistance, and increased atherogenic lipoprotein production.

Fed (post-prandial) conditions

The post-prandial state starts abruptly with calorie ingestion. Its duration is rather variable depending on meal size, glycemic index, and meal macronutrient composition. The metabolic changes of the fasting/post-prandial transition are mediated almost exclusively via insulin.

Whole-body post-prandial metabolism

Glucose. A typical meal might contain some 80 g of carbohydrate. The free glucose content of the body is around 12 g (assuming a plasma glucose concentration of 5 mmol/L and an extracellular fluid volume of 13 L). It follows that, as a result of a single meal, serum glucose concentrations might increase by around eightfold were there not an effective system for

buffering the effects of glucose and lipid ingestion. The prompt switch to
the post-prandial state mediated largely by insulin in healthy individuals
means that the blood glucose excursion is in fact usually limited to some
60% or less of the basal value. This is due principally to

1 rapid suppression of HGO
2 increased glucose disposal into cells for storage or metabolism

Both of these processes are typically abnormal in insulin resistance/T2DM.

Lipid. Extracellular triglyceride is confined to the plasma volume (approximately 3 L at a concentration of 1 mmol/L or 87.7 mg/dL), and the total
amount in circulation is therefore some 3 g. A typical meal might contain
enough triglyceride to increase this by a factor of around 10-fold. Again, in
healthy subjects, the typical excursion actually seen is of the order of 60%
of the basal value or less, largely as a result of insulin action in sensitive
individuals.

Skeletal muscle post-prandial metabolism

Glucose. Muscle switches rapidly from low to high glucose uptake under
the influence of insulin. The contribution of muscle to glucose disposal is
some 25–45% of the total oral load under normal conditions. Muscle
therefore sets the insulin sensitivity of insulin-dependent glucose disposal
for the whole body. Glucose is mostly stored, anaerobically metabolized to
lactate, or fully oxidized in the Krebs cycle via pyruvate. Insulin action
takes place via GLUT-4 translocation (enabling transport of glucose across
insulin-sensitive cell membranes) and via the regulation of glycogen
formation, glycolysis, and pyruvate oxidation.

Lipid. Lipid utilization decreases rapidly as glucose becomes available—
probably due to insulin suppression of NEFA release by adipose tissue, a
direct insulin effect in muscle and a concentration-dependent competition
between utilization of these two fuels (e.g., Randle cycle). TAG is cleared
by skeletal muscle and WAT, but the extent varies greatly, being higher in
endurance-trained athletes in whom TAG clearance is rapid and complete.
LPL is induced in muscle by training, and this variability has given rise to
the concept of inducible "fat tolerance."

Adipose tissue post-prandial metabolism

Adipose tissue normally contributes only around 5% to whole-body glucose
disposal, even in conditions of expanded adipose tissue mass. Glycogen
stores in adipose tissue are small, and glucose is therefore mainly taken
up for oxidative metabolism to generate ATP and to provide glycerol-
3-phosphate as a substrate for the esterification of FFAs into TAG. Free fatty
acid release from adipose tissue is prevented by insulin. The rate of NEFA
delivery to the liver is a major determinant of hepatic TAG secretion, and
reduced delivery is a major component of suppression of hepatic TAG

release by insulin *in vivo*. Reduced suppression of whole-body lipolysis in obesity is likely therefore to contribute to the dyslipidemia of the metabolic syndrome.

White adipose tissue (WAT) is therefore a "buffer" against the influx of dietary fatty acids into the circulation, just as the liver and muscle buffer the daily influx of glucose.

Adipose tissue extraction of chylomicron triglyceride following a meal is avid, clearing some 30% of arterial concentration in one passage through the tissue, the exact amount being highly variable from person to person. Defective action of adipose tissue LPL is associated with increased post-prandial lipemia.

Exercise

During light exercise (less than 25% VO$_2$max), there is little mobilization of muscle glycogen, but glucose uptake, oxidation, and conversion to lactate are increased. During heavier exercise (65% VO$_2$max), muscle glucose oxidation may increase by as much as 30-fold. Under these conditions, muscle glycogen breakdown occurs and lactate is produced as a result of anaerobic glycolysis and is recycled via the Cori cycle in the liver back to glucose for export to the exercising muscle. During a marathon, the mass of ATP turned over in skeletal muscle is roughly the same as the body mass of the individual.

The relative use of carbohydrate versus lipid as a metabolic fuel substrate varies with the intensity and duration of exercise and the fitness of the individual. Intramuscular TAG and muscle glycogen are depleted during exercise. GLUT-4 is stimulated by insulin and also by muscle contraction, leading to an increase in glucose uptake by some 10-fold. Free fatty acid utilization increases dramatically and is the major source of fuel in low-intensity exercise. At higher intensity, carbohydrate (CHO) becomes the predominant fuel source for the first 1–2 h followed by a switch to predominant lipid oxidation once glycogen becomes depleted. Brief, intense exercise in less-fit individuals tends to show CHO dependence, whereas rapid conversion to lipid metabolism is the hallmark of trained athletes. Individuals on low-fat diets show reduced fat oxidation and those on low-carbohydrate diets tend to demonstrate increased fat oxidation.

Summary

The tissues most involved in the uptake, storage, utilization, or release of macronutrients are skeletal muscle, adipose tissue, and the liver. Their function and ability to switch rapidly and completely between rest and exercise or between fasting and fed states are affected by obesity. The consequences of this metabolic inflexibility may extend from disordered metabolic fuel selection, particularly during exercise, to insulin resistance and development of the metabolic syndrome through the consequences of "lipotoxicity." Incomplete TAG clearance, sustained lipolysis, and a high-fat diet may contribute to the characteristic dyslipidemia of the metabolic syndrome.

Training and physical fitness tend to promote insulin sensitivity and more efficient extraction of glucose, FFAs, and TAG from the circulation and are associated with an early shift toward favoring fat over carbohydrate metabolism during exercise.

Pitfalls

- Not appreciating that exercise alone is rarely a successful strategy for weight loss without concurrent dietary modification.
- Allowing patients to give up on exercise when it does not produce rapid weight loss—at any given weight, it produces numerous health benefits in terms of lipid profile, insulin sensitivity, body composition, cardiovascular health, and general well-being and should therefore be promoted above and beyond its immediate effects in weight loss.
- Failing to take the opportunity to explain and tackle the physiological abnormalities seen in pre-diabetes, thus missing the opportunity to prevent or at least delay the onset of established T2DM.

Key web links

American Diabetes Association. http://www.diabetes.org/ [accessed on December 29, 2012].

Diabetes UK. http://www.diabetes.org.uk/ [accessed on December 29, 2012].

Nutrition.gov. http://www.nutrition.gov/ [accessed on December 29, 2012].

Centre for Disease Control. http://www.cdc.gov/diabetes/ [accessed on December 29, 2012].

NIDDK. http://www2.niddk.nih.gov/Research/ScientificAreas/Diabetes/MetabolismAnd IntegrativePhysiology/ADIP.htm [accessed on December 29, 2012].

Further reading

Church, T. (2011) Exercise in obesity, metabolic syndrome, and diabetes. *Progress in Cardiovascular Disease*, 53, 412–418.

Frayn, K.N., Karpe, F., Fielding, B.A., Macdonald, I.A. & Coppack, S.W. (2003) Integrative physiology of human adipose tissue. *International Journal of Obesity and Related Metabolic Disorder*, 27, 875–888.

Nelson, M.E., Rejeski, W.J., Blair, S.N. *et al.* (2007) Physical activity and public health in older adults: Recommendation from the American College of Sports Medicine and the American Heart Association. *Medicine and Science in Sports and Exercise*, 39, 1435–1445.

O'Donovan, G., Blazevich, A.J., Boreham, C. *et al.* (2010) The ABC of physical activity for health: A consensus statement from the British Association of Sport and Exercise Sciences. *Journal of Sports Science*, 28, 573–591.

Trayhurn, P., Drevon, C.A. & Eckel, J. (2011) Secreted proteins from adipose tissue and skeletal muscle – adipokines, myokines and adipose/muscle cross-talk. *Archives of Physiology and Biochemistry*, 117, 47–56.

Unger, R.H. (2002) Lipotoxic diseases. *Annual Review of Medicine*, 53, 319–336.

PART 2

Clinical Management of the Obese Individual

Robert Kushner, Section Editor

CHAPTER 6

Practical Guide to Clinical Assessment and Treatment Planning

---

Key points

- Optimal provision of obesity care in the office setting may require a "retooling" of office-based practices and functions.
- An obesity-focused history should address issues and concerns that will help formulate a weight loss plan specific to the patient. The conversation should be mutually respectful, express concern rather than judgment, be sensitive to the patient, and lessen stigma.
- Assessment of risk status due to overweight or obesity is based on the patient's BMI, waist circumference, and the existence of co-morbid conditions.

CASE STUDIES

Case study 1

DJ is a 26-year-old female who presents as a new patient. She has been in good health and is on no medications. Her weight history is notable for being overweight since childhood, weighing 160 lb in high school, 180 lb in college, and increasing to 220 lb over the past 4 years. She attributes her weight gain to enjoying fast foods, eating out often with friends, and leading a sedentary lifestyle. She also binges weekly when she is alone at night. She is single and rarely cooks. DJ is ready to engage in active weight loss since her weight is hindering her social life. The physical examination is unremarkable and her waist circumference is 92 cm. At 5'9", her calculated BMI is 32.6 kg/m², or class I obesity. Her elevated waist circumference places her in the very-high-risk category. Fasting laboratory values are normal.

Comment: A weight loss treatment plan is formulated using convenient low-calorie meal replacements, setting a goal of increasing daily steps, and referral to a health psychologist to address her binge behavior.

Practical Manual of Clinical Obesity, First Edition. Robert Kushner, Victor Lawrence and Sudhesh Kumar.
© 2013 John Wiley & Sons, Ltd. Published 2013 by John Wiley & Sons, Ltd.

Case study 2

JH is a 48-year-old male who makes an appointment today concerned about a 30-lb weight gain over the past 4 years: 20lb was gained after quitting cigarette smoking and another 10lb was gained after he changed from an active to a sedentary job. He has no routine eating schedule, frequently skips meals, and does not exercise. He is married with two children and is stressed due to tight finances. On examination, his height is 5'10" and weight 250lb. His calculated BMI is 36 kg/m² and BP 140/88, and he has a large abdominal pannus. Laboratory values notable for elevated fasting glucose of 116 mg/dL, triglyceride 280 mg/dL, and HDL cholesterol 36 mg/dL are consistent with the metabolic syndrome.

Comment: Primary treatment is weight loss. JH was referred to a registered dietitian for medical nutrition counseling and a medical follow-up in 2 months.

Setting up a clinic

Although not legally considered a disability, patients with obesity may have special needs that should be recognized and responded to. This may require "retooling" the office to accommodate the increased weight and size of this patient population, having counseling tools readily accessible in the examination room, and educating the office staff about the need to exhibit a non-judgmental and empathetic attitude toward obese patients. The following checklist can be used to audit the office setting:

- Sturdy open-arm chairs and firm sofas in the waiting room that can support increased body size and weight.
- Availability of a scale that measures in excess of 350lb (169kg). The weight scale should preferably have a wide base with a nearby handle bar for support if necessary. To protect privacy, consider placing the scale in a private area of the office to avoid unnecessary embarrassment. A wall-mounted sliding statiometer to measure height or a firm height meter attached to the scale should also be available. Accurate measurement of height is necessary to calculate BMI.
- A flexible tape measure for assessment of waist circumference.
- Examination rooms should have large gowns available to wear as well as a sturdy step stool to mount the examination tables. In addition to the standard adult size, each room should be equipped with large adult and thigh blood pressure cuffs for measurement of blood pressure. A bladder cuff that is not the appropriate width for the patient's arm circumference will cause a systematic error in blood pressure measurement.
- Availability of handouts that are readily accessible to assist in patient risk assessment, tracking of diet and physical activity, counseling materials, Internet sites, and referral resources.

Broaching the topic of obesity

Broaching the topic of body weight and obesity is very difficult for many physicians. Part of the difficulty lies in time restraints during a busy practice, lack of effective treatment options, inadequate reimbursement, and low confidence or insufficient training in weight management counseling. Furthermore, for many physicians, discussion of body weight does not occur due to not knowing how to raise a sensitive issue, fear of insulting the patient, and attitudes or biases that are particular to obesity. There are few other conditions in medical practice and in our society that are as stigmatized and shunned as obesity. Some view obesity as a personal moral failure, while others believe it is solely due to sloth and gluttony. Others feel that it is a personal responsibility to be solved by the patient alone. In reality, obesity is a complex disease due to genetic, biological, economic, environmental, psychosocial, and behavioral determinants. Rather than blaming patients for their weight, recognizing obesity as a medical condition will pave the way for a frank, open, and respectful dialogue.

There is no clearly established method for telling patients they are overweight or obese. However, initiating talk about weight is an interactive process, with information sharing between patient and physician. The initial goals of the conversation are to inform the patient of his or her body weight related to health standards, clearly convey the health risks associated with excess weight, explore the patient's motivation and readiness to engage in weight control, elicit barriers to behavior change, and establish practical lifestyle changes and short-term goals. When first raising the topic about body weight, words matter. The approach physicians use to broach this potentially sensitive topic may influence how patients react emotionally and cognitively to the discussion and advice provided. Language used by the physician sets the stage for the interaction. It is up to the physician to decide which words will be most constructive and therapeutic. The reason for the concern is that the word *obesity* is a highly charged emotive term. It has a significant pejorative meaning with many patients, leaving them feeling judged and blamed when labeled as obese. The bottom line is that the physician and patient must use shared terminology that is agreeable, inoffensive, and understandable to both individuals. The conversation should be mutually respectful, express concern rather than judgment, be sensitive to the patient, and lessen stigma.

Taking an obesity-focused history

The first step in initiating obesity care is to take a comprehensive history that addresses issues and concerns specific to obesity treatment. This

---

Box 6.1 Etiological factors for weight gain identified from history

Physiological
  Genetic (heritability)
  Pregnancy
  Menopause
  Weight-gaining medications
  Smoking cessation
  Endocrine disorders: polycystic ovary syndrome (PCOS), hypothyroidism, Cushing
    disease
Behavioral
  Dietary
    Unhealthy eating patterns, grazing, nibbling, mindless eating, large volume
      consumption of high-energy foods and beverages
  BED, bulimia nervosa
  Physical activity
    Reduced leisure time activity
    Increased sedentary behaviors
    Insufficient moderate- and vigorous-intensity exercise
    Development of physical limitations to exercise

---

obesity-focused history allows the physician to develop tailored treatment recommendations that are more consistent with the needs and goals of the individual patient. Information from the history should address the factors that contributed to the patient's obesity, the effect of obesity on the patient's health, the patient's risk for developing and/or the presence of obesity-related co-morbidities, the patient's goals and expectations regarding treatment, and the patient's motivation and interest in engaging in a weight management program. Box 6.1 lists etiological causes of weight gain. Two contributing factors, the presence of endocrinological disorders and the use of weight-gaining medications, need to be addressed as treatment of the disorder and substitution for another medication, respectively, will impact the patient's weight.

The psychosocial history provides the most important information for formulating a tailored and implementable treatment plan. Take time to assess the patient's contextual living conditions. For example, knowing whether the patient lives alone or with others, the amount of social support available, if he is employed, works from home or from an office, is time pressured or has flexibility, is under financial hardship or is experiencing a great deal of stress will be important in devising a counseling plan. Assessment of dietary and physical activity behaviors is addressed in later chapters. The psychological/psychiatric history should particularly assess for the presence of mood and anxiety disorders. Persons with severe obesity are almost five times more likely to have experienced an episode of major depression in the past year as compared to average-weight individuals. This relationship appears to be stronger for women than men. Mild forms of depression, or those related to the patient's current body weight, can frequently be treated simultaneously with weight management. The occurrence of a major depressive episode, however, will likely interfere with the treatment of obesity.

Body image is an important aspect of quality of life (QOL) for many individuals. Body image dissatisfaction is common in overweight and obese individuals, and the degree of dissatisfaction seems to be directly related to the amount of excess weight a person has. Two eating disorders, *binge eating disorder (BED)*—consumption of an objectively large amount of food in a brief period of time (e.g., 2 h) with the patient's report of subjective loss of control during the overeating episode—and *bulimia nervosa*—binge eating with loss of control, which is accompanied by compensatory behaviors including vomiting, laxative abuse, or excessive exercise—need to be evaluated and warrant treatment independent of weight reduction. Persons with an active substance abuse disorder and those with an active psychosis are inappropriate for weight loss treatment.

Physical examination of the obese patient

Assessment of risk status due to overweight or obesity is based on the patient's BMI, waist circumference, and the existence of co-morbid conditions. Actual measurement of weight and height is an important first step in the identification of an at-risk individual and during re-evaluation. Small amounts of weight gain will likely be missed if the patient is not weighed. To protect privacy, consideration should be given to placing the scale in a private area of the office to avoid unnecessary embarrassment. BMI is calculated as weight (kg)/height (m)^2 or as weight (lb)/height (in.)^2 × 703. A BMI table is more conveniently used for simple reference (see Figure 6.1). BMI is recommended since it provides an estimate of body fat and is related to risk of disease. An internationally accepted classification of obesity based on BMI is presented in Table 6.1.

In addition to BMI, the risk of overweight and obesity is independently associated with excess abdominal fat and fitness level. Population studies have shown that people with large waist circumferences have impaired health and increased cardiovascular risk compared to those with normal waist circumferences within the healthy, overweight, and class I obesity BMI categories. The threshold for excessive abdominal fat varies according to guidelines and ethnicity. Ethnicity-specific values for waist circumference defined by the International Diabetes Federation (IDF) are shown in

BMI	19	20	21	22	23	24	25	26	27	28	29	30	31	32	33	34	35
Height (inches)							**Body weight (pounds)**										
58	91	96	100	105	110	115	119	124	129	134	138	143	148	153	158	162	167
59	94	99	104	109	114	119	124	128	133	138	143	148	153	158	163	168	173
60	97	102	107	112	118	123	128	133	138	143	148	153	158	163	168	174	179
61	100	106	111	116	122	127	132	137	143	148	153	158	164	169	174	180	185
62	104	109	115	120	126	131	136	142	147	153	158	164	169	175	180	186	191
63	107	113	118	124	130	135	141	146	152	158	163	169	175	180	186	191	197
64	110	116	122	128	134	140	145	151	157	163	169	174	180	186	192	197	204
65	114	120	126	132	138	144	150	156	162	168	174	180	186	192	198	204	210
66	118	124	130	136	142	148	155	161	167	173	179	186	192	198	204	210	216
67	121	127	134	140	146	153	159	166	172	178	185	191	198	204	211	217	223
68	125	131	138	144	151	158	164	171	177	184	190	197	203	210	216	223	230
69	128	135	142	149	155	162	169	176	182	189	196	203	209	216	223	230	236
70	132	139	146	153	160	167	174	181	188	195	202	209	216	222	229	236	243
71	136	143	150	157	165	172	179	186	193	200	208	215	222	229	236	243	250
72	140	147	154	162	169	177	184	191	199	206	213	221	228	235	242	250	258
73	144	151	159	166	174	182	189	197	204	212	219	227	235	242	250	257	265
74	148	155	163	171	179	186	194	202	210	218	225	233	241	249	256	264	272
75	152	160	168	176	184	192	200	208	216	224	232	240	248	256	264	272	279
76	156	164	172	180	189	197	205	213	221	230	238	246	254	263	271	279	287

BMI	36	37	38	39	40	41	42	43	44	45	46	47	48	49	50	51	52	53	54
58	172	177	181	186	191	196	201	205	210	215	220	224	229	234	239	244	248	253	258
59	178	183	188	193	198	203	208	212	217	222	227	232	237	242	247	252	257	262	267
60	184	189	194	199	204	209	215	220	225	230	235	240	245	250	255	261	266	271	276
61	190	195	201	206	211	217	222	227	232	238	243	248	254	259	264	269	275	280	285
62	196	202	207	213	218	224	229	235	240	246	251	256	262	267	273	278	284	289	295
63	203	208	214	220	225	231	237	242	248	254	259	265	270	278	282	287	293	299	304
64	209	215	221	227	232	238	244	250	256	262	267	273	279	285	291	296	302	308	314
65	216	222	228	234	240	246	252	258	264	270	276	282	288	294	300	306	312	318	324
66	223	229	235	241	247	253	260	266	272	278	284	291	297	303	309	315	322	328	334
67	230	236	242	249	255	261	268	274	280	287	293	299	306	312	319	325	331	338	344
68	236	243	249	256	262	269	276	282	289	295	302	308	315	322	328	335	341	348	354
69	243	250	257	263	270	277	284	291	297	304	311	318	324	331	338	345	351	358	365
70	250	257	264	271	278	285	292	299	306	313	320	327	334	341	348	355	362	369	376
71	257	265	272	279	286	293	301	308	315	322	329	338	343	351	358	365	372	379	386
72	265	272	279	287	294	302	309	316	324	331	338	346	353	361	368	375	383	390	397
73	272	280	288	295	302	310	318	325	333	340	348	355	363	371	378	386	393	401	408
74	280	287	295	303	311	319	326	334	342	350	358	365	373	381	389	396	404	412	420
75	287	295	303	311	319	327	335	343	351	359	367	375	383	391	399	407	415	423	431
76	295	304	312	320	328	336	344	353	361	369	377	385	394	402	410	418	426	435	443

Figure 6.1 BMI table.

Table 6.1 Classification of overweight and obesity by BMI, waist circumference, and associated disease risk[a].

Disease risk[a] (relative to normal weight and waist circumference)

	BMI (kg/m²)	Obesity class	Men ≤ 40 in. (≤102 cm)	>40 in. (>102 cm)
			Women ≤ 35 in. (≤88 cm)	>35 in. (>88 cm)
Underweight	<18.5		–	–
Normal	18.5–24.9		–	–
Overweight	25.0–29.9		Increased	High
Obesity	30.0–34.9	I	High	Very high
	35.0–39.9	II	Very high	Very high
Extreme obesity	≥40	III	Extremely high	Extremely high

Reproduced from NHLBI Obesity Education Initiative. (2000) *The Practical Guide: Identification, Evaluation, and Treatment of Overweight and Obesity in Adults*. NIH Publication No. 00-4084, October. US Department of Health and Human Services, Public Health Service, National Institutes of Health, National Heart, Lung, and Blood Institute.
[a] Disease risk for T2DM, hypertension, and CVD.

Table 6.2 Ethnicity-specific values for waist circumference.

Ethnic group	Waist circumference
Europeans	
Men	>94 cm (37 in.)
Women	>80 cm (31.5 in.)
South Asians and Chinese	
Men	>90 cm (35 in.)
Women	>80 cm (31.5 in.)
Japanese	
Men	>85 cm (33.5 in.)
Women	>90 cm (35 in.)
Ethnic South and Central Americans	Use South Asian data until more specific data are available
Sub-Saharan Africans	Use European data until more specific data are available
Eastern Mediterranean and Middle East (Arab)	Use European data until more specific data are available

Reproduced from Albertiet *et al.Lancet* 2005, 366, 1059.

Table 6.2. Measurement of abdominal girth is not a difficult procedure and only takes a few seconds. Overweight persons with waist circumferences exceeding the limits defined by IDF should be urged more strongly to pursue weight reduction since it categorically increases disease risk for each BMI class. The importance of measuring and documenting waist circumference in patients with a BMI less than $35 \, \text{kg/m}^2$ is due to the independent contribution of abdominal fat to the development of co-morbid diseases, particularly the metabolic syndrome.

Determination of fitness level is another modifier to assessing risk associated with BMI. High cardiorespiratory fitness is associated with lower levels of whole-body and abdominal obesity for a given BMI. Longitudinal studies have shown that cardiorespiratory fitness (as measured by a maximal treadmill exercise test) is an important predictor of all-cause mortality independent of BMI and body composition. These observations highlight the importance of taking an exercise history during the assessment as well as emphasizing the incorporation of moderately vigorous physical activity as a treatment approach.

Box 6.2 Obesity-related organ systems review

Cardiovascular

Hypertension

Congestive heart failure (CHF)

Cor pulmonale

Varicose veins

Pulmonary embolism

Coronary artery disease

Endocrine

Metabolic syndrome

T2DM

Dyslipidemia

PCOS/androgenicity

Amenorrhea/infertility/menstrual disorders

Musculo-skeletal

Hyperuricemia and gout

Immobility

Osteoarthritis (knees and hips)

Low back pain

Psychological

Depression/low self-esteem

Body image disturbance

Social stigmatization

Integument

Striae distensae (stretch marks)

Stasis pigmentation of legs

Lymphedema

Cellulitis

Intertrigo, carbuncles

Acanthosis nigricans/skin tags

Respiratory

Dyspnea

Obstructive sleep apnea (OSA)

Hypoventilation syndrome

Pickwickian syndrome

Asthma

Gastro-intestinal (GI)

Gastroesophageal reflux disease (GERD)

NAFLD

Cholelithiasis

Hernias

Colon cancer

Genitourinary

Urinary stress incontinence

Obesity-related glomerulopathy

Hypogonadism (male)

Breast and uterine cancer

Pregnancy complications

Neurologic

Stroke

Idiopathic intracranial hypertension

Meralgia paresthetica

Identifying the high-risk obese patient

Patients at very high absolute risk that trigger the need for intense risk factor modification and management include the following: established coronary heart disease; presence of other atherosclerotic diseases, such as peripheral arterial disease, abdominal aortic aneurysm, or symptomatic carotid artery disease; T2DM; and sleep apnea. Presence of the metabolic syndrome should also prompt urgent treatment. Other symptoms and diseases that are directly or indirectly related to obesity are listed in Box 6.2. Although individuals will vary, the number and severity of organ-specific co-morbid conditions usually rise with increasing levels of obesity. Even though many of these conditions may not be life threatening, they are often the chief concern and determine the QOL for the patient and, therefore, should trigger active obesity treatment.

There is no single laboratory test or diagnostic evaluation that is indicated for all patients with obesity. The specific evaluation performed should be based on the presentation of symptoms, risk factors, and index of suspicion. However, based on several other screening guideline recommendations, most, if not all, patients should have a fasting lipid panel (total, LDL, and HDL cholesterol and triglyceride levels) and blood glucose measured at presentation along with blood pressure determination.

Pitfalls

- Patients who are obese will care if the seats in the waiting room cannot accommodate them, the scale cannot weigh them, or the gown is too small to fit them.
- If physicians wait for patients to bring up their weight problem prior to initiating weight loss counseling, then many missed opportunities will occur to provide obesity care.
- Initiating weight loss treatment for obesity is dependent on the patient's weight history or psychosocial background: all treatment recommendations are not the same.

Key web links

Clinical Guidelines on the Identification, Evaluation, and Treatment of Overweight and Obesity in Adults. http://www.nhlbi.nih.gov/guidelines/obesity/index.htm [accessed on December 29, 2012].

Assessment and management of adult obesity. Evaluating your patients for overweight or obesity. Booklet 2. American Medical Association. http://www.ama-assn.org/resources/doc/public-health/booklet2.pdf [accessed on December 29, 2012].

Logue, J., Thompson, L., Romanes, F. *et al.* (2010) Management of obesity: Summary of SIGN guidelines. *BMJ*, 340, 474–477. http://www.sign.ac.uk/guidelines/fulltext/115/index.html [accessed on December 29, 2012].

Further reading

Appel, L.J., Clark, J.M., Yeh, H.C. *et al.* (2011) Comparative effectiveness of weight-loss interventions in clinical practice. *New England Journal of Medicine*, 365, 1959–1968.

Dutton, G.R., Tan, F., Perri, M.G. *et al.* (2010) What words should we use when discussing excess weight? *Journal of the American Board of Family Medicine*, 23, 606–613.

Kushner, R.F. (2010) Tackling obesity. Is primary care up to the challenge? Commentary. *Archives of Internal Medicine*, 170, 121–123.

LeBlanc, E.S., O'connor, E., Whitlock, E.P., Patnode, C.D. & Kapka, T. (2011) Effectiveness of primary care-relevant treatments for obesity in adults: A systematic review for the U.S. preventive services task force. *Annals of Internal Medicine*, 155, 434–447.

Robert, E., Post, R.E., Mainous, A.G. *et al.* (2011) The influence of physician acknowledgment of patients' weight status on patient perceptions of overweight and obesity in the United States. *Archives of Internal Medicine*, 171, 316–321.

Silk, A.W. & McTigue, K.M. (2011) Reexamining the physical examination for obese patients. *Journal of American Medical Association*, 305, 193–194.

Tsai, A.G. & Wadden, T.A. (2009) Treatment of obesity in primary care practice in the United States: A systematic review. *Journal of General Internal Medicine*, 24, 1073–1079.

Wadden, T.A., Volger, S., Sarwer, D.B. *et al.* (2011) A two-year randomized trial of obesity treatment in primary care practice. *New England Journal of Medicine*, 365, 1969–1979.

CHAPTER 7

Stages of Obesity and Weight Maintenance

Key points
- The initial treatment goal is to achieve approximately 10% loss of body weight.
- Weight stability or a plateau occurs when reduced caloric intake matches a reduced energy expenditure.
- There are multiple behavioral, physiological, and metabolic adaptations that make weight loss maintenance difficult to sustain.
- A successful weight maintainer leads an active life, has flexible control over eating behavior with a regular meal rhythm, and uses positive coping mechanisms.

CASE STUDIES

Case study 1

BB is a 29-year-old female with a BMI of 38 kg/m² who presents for weight management. As part of your initial evaluation, you ask her to recall her weight and associated life events since high school. She reveals a pattern of frequent and significant weight cycling, with weight losses ranging from 11 to 18 kg by following meal delivery programs, commercial weight loss programs, and multiple self-imposed diets. She states that she is an "all-or-nothing" dieter and finds it hard to do anything in moderation, including her professional and volunteer work. She also discloses that she suffers from mood swings that tend to correspond with her weight fluctuations.

Comment: You inform BB that she would benefit from seeing a health psychologist for further psychological and behavioral evaluation and counsel her on the need for consistency in her diet and physical activity. You recommend a moderate reduction in calories and ask her to track her diet. A follow-up visit is arranged.

Case study 2

NA is a 53-year-old female who presented with a BMI of 31 kg/m². By following a lifestyle modification program of caloric reduction and physical activity, she has lost 8% of her body weight over 6 months. She returns to the office frustrated after reaching a weight plateau for several months, complaining that "the diet isn't working anymore."

Practical Manual of Clinical Obesity, First Edition. Robert Kushner, Victor Lawrence and Sudhesh Kumar.
© 2013 John Wiley & Sons, Ltd. Published 2013 by John Wiley & Sons, Ltd.

Comment: After reviewing her diet and physical activity patterns, you explain that stabilization of her weight implies that her caloric intake exactly matches her caloric expenditure and that her muscles have become more efficient doing the same exercises. To achieve a new "calorie gap," you ask her to track her caloric intake to ensure increased adherence to the dietary goal, recommend resistance training exercises to increase lean body mass, and to vary her aerobic exercises to utilize different muscle groups. You also reassure her that she is doing a good job and to continue the healthy behaviors.

For many patients, obesity is a chronic lifelong disorder and therefore may present to the clinician in one of many stages: desiring initial weight loss, frustrated at a weight loss plateau, satisfied at weight maintenance, or distraught about weight regain. Each stage presents a set of challenges and opportunities for the patient and clinician. This chapter reviews the definitions and factors that are unique to each stage.

Stages of obesity

Weight loss
A conversation about weight loss may be initiated by the clinician or patient. The initial goal is to achieve approximately 10% loss of body weight. If this target is achieved, consideration may be given for further weight reduction. For most patients, this is a practical and realistic goal. Outcome studies have shown that a 5–10% weight loss is enough to achieve significant improvement in obesity-associated metabolic risk factors, with improved glycemic control and reduced blood pressure and cholesterol levels. Besides the positive health benefits of a lower body weight, beneficial effects on psychosocial functioning and mental aspects of QOL have also been demonstrated. With a reduced body weight, fewer obstacles are perceived concerning activities such as social gatherings, buying clothes, going away for holidays, bathing in public, and having intimate relations with a partner. Mental aspects of QOL, such as mental well-being, are also positively related to a reduced body weight.

Weight loss patterns
Initial weight loss has been identified as a predictor for later weight loss and for weight loss maintenance. The greater the initial weight loss, the better is the subsequent outcome. Initial weight loss can reflect better adherence with the treatment regimen. It is still unclear precisely how the early weight loss response predicts long-term outcome and how it should be defined. The longer the weight loss has been maintained, the better are the chances for further continuation of a lower body weight. Subjects who

have maintained weight losses for a longer time report that they use less effort in continued weight control.

Weight loss plateau

Irrespective of treatment, whether diet, exercise, behavior modification, or pharmacotherapy, most, although not quite all, treatment programs result in continuous weight loss for about 6 months, after which weight loss plateaus. Thus, whatever method is being used, strategies have to change from the first weight loss period to the maintenance phase. Reassurance, support, and acceptance are important components of the treatment, so that the patient understands and hopefully accepts that further weight loss may not take place easily. The plateau can easily be explained on physiological grounds. With the reduction in lean body mass, which is an inevitable consequence of any weight loss, the BMR will go down and the overall needs of the individual after weight loss become lesser. Thus, intake and expenditure will balance at a lower level after successful weight loss, and when this takes place, no further weight loss can be expected. Continued weight loss will require further reduction in caloric intake and/or increased caloric expenditure.

Weight loss maintenance

Weight loss maintenance implies keeping a weight loss accomplished by treatment interventions or by the patient's own efforts. The specific criteria used, however, differ. Examples of definitions are "achieving an intentional weight loss of at least 10% of initial body weight and maintaining this body weight for at least 1 year" or "losing at least 5% of baseline body weight between baseline and follow-up and maintaining that weight or less for a further 2 years." Maintenance of weight loss is extremely challenging and is thought to be due to several factors, including life events, recidivism of behaviors, and physiological and metabolic adaptations.

Weight cycling

Weight cycling refers to the repeated loss and regain of weight. Although many patients believe that such swings in body weight make you fatter, weight cycling, whether natural or experimental, does not result in permanent alterations of body composition or resting energy expenditure nor in the alteration of fat mobilization. However, weight cycling still remains a problem from the psychological point of view, as it may be associated with a number of negative factors related to eating behavior. Weight cycling has sometimes been associated with mental distress and psychopathology; however, mental distress could also characterize the person as being more prone to diet and having more difficulties in sustaining the weight lost, rather than it being a consequence of the weight cycling. More disturbed eating behaviors and a higher prevalence of binge eating have also been noted among weight cyclers. The greater the number of weight loss efforts, the greater was the occurrence or severity of binge eating. However, whether weight cycling causes binge eating or vice versa could not be resolved from these studies.

Factors affecting weight loss maintenance

Physical activity

Maintaining weight loss is the greatest challenge for patients. Physical activity is related to long-term weight maintenance in most studies. Physical activity can help weight maintenance through direct energy expenditure and by improved physical fitness, which facilitates the amount and intensity of daily activities. Physical activity can also improve well-being, which may in turn facilitate other positive behaviors needed for weight maintenance. Walking is one of the most frequent aspects of physical exercise reported by patients. A higher number of pedometer-recorded daily steps and other measures, including everyday activities, have likewise been found among weight maintainers. Impaired physical functioning in daily life, implying limitations in the ability for ambulation, has correspondingly predicted later weight relapse. Perceiving barriers in the life situation for carrying out physical activity has also been related to poorer weight maintenance, whereas confidence concerning exercise may promote long-term weight management.

Dietary intake

Weight loss maintenance is associated with lower total caloric intake and reduced portion sizes. More specifically, it is also associated with reduced frequency of snacks and less dietary fat. Reduction of particular food types, such as fried foods like French fries, dairy products like cheese and butter, sweets, meat, high-fat snacks, and desserts, has also been seen in persons successfully maintaining their weight. The importance of including high-quality foods, such as fruits and vegetables, and healthy eating has also been noted. Change toward a more regular meal rhythm has been identified as helpful in long-term weight loss, and regularly eating breakfast has been reported more often among weight maintainers. It is suggested that breakfast can reduce hunger, making the breakfast eaters choose less-energy-dense foods during the rest of the day as well as giving better energy to perform physical activity during the day.

Physiological factors

In addition to behavioral factors, there are several physiological and metabolic adaptations that make weight loss maintenance difficult to achieve.

Resting and non-resting metabolic rates decrease as individuals lose weight. This is due to a reduction in lean body mass, compensatory changes in energy expenditure, muscle efficiency during physical activity, and drop in leptin. These are presumably evolutionary defense mechanisms to combat starvation and weight loss.

The successful weight maintainer

To summarize the findings on factors affecting weight loss maintenance, a profile characterizing the "successful weight maintainer" can be suggested. This ideal person starts losing weight successfully quite early in treatment and reaches the self-determined weight loss goals. Our ideal weight maintainer leads an active life with less television watching and does more leisure activities, such as walking and cycling. He or she is in control over eating behavior and is not overly disturbed by hunger. Food intake is kept at a lower level; meal rhythm is regular, always including breakfast; and healthy foods are chosen. Snacking is reduced. When cravings occur, they can be dealt with by various mechanisms. If experiencing a relapse, our weight maintainer can handle this in a balanced way without exaggerating it as a detrimental failure. Controls are flexible rather than rigid, and there is self-sufficiency and autonomy.

Although personality findings are sparse in the research on weight loss, some conclusions can be inferred from the overall findings in the literature. Strengths include a capacity for control and flexible thinking and also the ability to cope with relapse rather than reverting to a more dichotomous, all-or-none thinking. The ability to create and sustain a meal structure and alter food habits can also imply psychological resources and capacities. Finding coping strategies to handle cravings and stressful situations in life reflects an ability to use creativity and thinking to come up with one's own solutions. Self-monitoring suggests self-awareness, and self-sufficiency and autonomy would likewise constitute strengths. Not surprisingly, this ideal weight maintainer has fewer inner afflictions and instability, such as mental distress, binge eating, and weight cycling, but instead more stability of weight patterns, eating, and emotions. Support is provided by the social context, although our weight maintainer may prefer to rely on their own solutions. There may be more of an internal motivation for weight loss, with wishes to become more confident and feel better about oneself. A healthy narcissism, implying there is at least some energy invested in oneself, with caring for oneself, one's appearance, and physical status, can also be considered a strength.

For a list of factors associated with weight regain and weight loss maintenance, see Box 7.1 and Box 7.2, respectively.

Box 7.1 Suggested factors associated with weight regain

Failure to reach a self-determined weight goal

Attribution of obesity to medical factors
Sedentary lifestyle
Disinhibited eating
More hunger
Binge eating
Eating in response to negative emotions and stress
Depression
Distress
Poor coping strategies
Escape-avoidance to problem
Passive wishes
Help seeking
Motivation for weight loss: medical reasons, other persons
Personality traits indicating more disturbances

Box 7.2 Suggested factors associated with weight loss maintenance.

Achievement of the self-determined weight loss goal

More initial weight loss
Physically active lifestyle
Regular meal rhythm
Eating breakfast
Less dietary fat, more healthy foods
Reduced frequency of snacks
Flexible control over eating
Self-monitoring
Better coping strategies
Ability to find ways to handle craving
Self-efficacy
Autonomy
"Healthy narcissism"
Motivation for weight loss: becoming more confident

Pitfalls
- Not establishing clear, practical, and achievable goals for weight loss will lead patients to be frustrated, disappointed, and confused.
- Assuming that patients can "break through" a weight plateau simply by eating less food and "trying harder" ignores the physiological and metabolic factors that contribute to weight stability.
- Inattention to the patient's environmental, social, and psychological factors and personality will hinder counseling for long-term weight maintenance.

Further reading

Appelhans, B.M., Whited, M.C., Schneider, K.L. & Pagoto, S.L. (2011) Time to abandon the notion of personal choice in dietary counseling for obesity. *Journal of the American Dietetic Association*, 111, 1130–1136.

Bond, D.S., Phelan, S., Leahey, T.M., Hill, J.O. & Wing, R.R. (2009) Weight-loss maintenance in successful weight losers: Surgical vs non-surgical methods. *International Journal of Obesity*, 33, 173–180.

Elfhag, K. & Rossner, S. (2005) Who succeeds in maintaining weight loss? A conceptual review of factors associated with weight loss maintenance and weight regain. *Obesity Reviews*, 6, 67–85.

Kushner, R.F. & Choi, S.W. (2010) Prevalence of unhealthy lifestyle patterns among overweight and obese adults. *Obesity*, 18, 1160–1167.

LeBlanc, E.S., O'connor, E., Whitlock, E.P., Patnode, C.D. & Kapka, T. (2011) Effectiveness of primary care-relevant treatments for obesity in adults: A systematic review for the U.S. preventive services task force. *Annals of Internal Medicine*, 155, 434–447.

Pinto, A.M., Gorin, A.A., Raynor, H.A., Tate, D.F., Fava, J.L. & Wing, R.R. (2008) Successful weight-loss maintenance in relation to method of weight loss. *Obesity*, 16, 2456–2461.

Teixeira, P.J., Going, S.B., Sarkinha, L.B. & Lohman, T.G. (2005) A review of psychological pre-treatment predictors of weight control. *Obesity Reviews*, 6, 43–65.

Teixeira, P.J., Going, S.B., Houtkooper, L.B. *et al.* (2006) Pretreatment predictors of attrition and successful weight management in women. *International Journal of Obesity*, 28, 1124–1133.

Westenhoefer, J., von Falck, B., Stellfeldt, A. & Fintelmann, S. (2004) Behavioral correlates of successful weight reduction over 3 y. Results from the Lean Habits Study. *International Journal of Obesity*, 28, 334–335.

CHAPTER 8

Dietary Management

Key points

- Body weight change is primarily dependent on caloric deficit, not the macronutrient composition of the diet.
- A diet history can be quickly and conveniently assessed by taking a 24-h recall or asking the patient to complete a food journal.
- Dietary counseling should address the patient's eating patterns. This involves the distribution of food, portion sizes, timing, and speed of eating.
- An initial goal is to help patients achieve a structured and planned eating schedule.
- Use of meal replacement products, low-energy-dense foods, and very-low-calorie diets may be useful strategies.

CASE STUDIES

Case study 1

NG is a 52-year-old man with hypertension and obesity and a BMI of 35 kg/m². Dietary management and weight reduction are indicated, and the patient agrees to focus on his diet as the first step. After taking a 24-h recall, you learn that NG consumes convenient foods that are high in calories and fat. He skips breakfast and his lunch and dinner are large and typically do not include fruits and vegetables.
Comment: As a first step, you ask him to use a meal replacement bar for breakfast, "down size" his food portions at lunch and dinner, include a vegetable and fruit with each meal, slow down his eating, and begin to look at the caloric content of his food choices. You also ask him to track his diet using a smart phone application.

Case study 2

LC is a 29-year-old female with a BMI of 39 kg/m² who presents after losing 10 kg by following a very-low-carbohydrate popular diet for 2 months. Although happy with the weight loss, she complains of constipation and a bad taste in her mouth. She finds the diet easy to follow since she has eliminated all starches, fruits, and most vegetables. Her protein sources are whole dairy products, luncheon meats, and eggs. A lipid panel is obtained which shows total cholesterol 280 mg/dL, LDL cholesterol 175 mg/dL, triglyceride 105 mg/dL, and HDL cholesterol 45 mg/dL.

Practical Manual of Clinical Obesity, First Edition. Robert Kushner, Victor Lawrence and Sudhesh Kumar.
© 2013 John Wiley & Sons, Ltd. Published 2013 by John Wiley & Sons, Ltd.

> **Comment**: Based on her symptoms and lipid panel results, you recommend that she adds more vegetables and whole grains to her diet and chooses leaner sources of protein such as skimmed dairy products, poultry, lean meats, beans, and legumes. You also educate her about the importance of including multiple food groups and nutrients in her diet.

Box 8.1 IOM report on acceptable macronutrient levels in the diet.

- 45–65% of total calories from carbohydrates
- 20–35% of total calories from fat
- 10–35% of total calories from protein

Dietary treatment for obesity

Dietary counseling for weight loss is the most important component of the treatment plan for obesity. Weight loss is primarily dependent on reducing total caloric intake, not the proportions of carbohydrate, fat, and protein in the diet. The macronutrient composition (i.e., proportion of calories from carbohydrate, fat, and protein) will ultimately be determined by the patient's taste preferences, cooking style, culture, and food purchases. As a general guide, the IOM report published in 2002 recommends a broad range of acceptable macronutrient levels (Box 8.1).

Caloric (energy) deficit diet can be achieved by many means. A 2–4 MJ (500–1000 kcal) deficit from daily intake (i.e., from intakes that are weight maintaining, rather than weight increasing) results in an approximately 0.5–1 kg weight loss per week. This is a practical and achievable goal for most patients. Since it is difficult to accurately measure the patient's true caloric intake, it is oftentimes more beneficial to focus on the number of calories that the patient should subtract from their habitual diet in order to lose weight. Nonetheless, the first step in dietary counseling is to assess the patient's current diet to identify targets of opportunity for change.

Assessing food intake

The first step is to understand the patient's current daily food *choices* and *portions*. There are two commonly used tools for assessing a patient's eating behaviors, each having their own advantages and disadvantages: typical day recall and food journal. Each of these tools is affected by under-reporting bias but does serve the purpose of assessing basic dietary patterns.

1 A typical day recall or 24-h recall begins with an open-ended question such as "I'd like to learn more about your diet. Can you tell me what you eat and drink in a typical day, starting with the first thing in the morning and ending when you go to sleep at night?" This non-

judgmental approach is important because it allows patients to reveal their dietary patterns without guilt or embarrassment. When using a typical day recall, remember to prompt patients to provide details such as timing and location of eating and snacking, specific food choices and portions, beverages consumed, and environmental and emotional triggers for eating. One could also ask about weekday and weekend variations as weekdays are often more structured and lower in high-energy foods than weekends. Another useful question is "Do you normally lose weight or gain weight when on holiday?" The answers to this question can then be used in helping the patient identify triggers for overeating and alter behaviors to reduce food intake at home. For example, the patient may have reduced their intake as they tend not to overeat with other people around, or perhaps they were preoccupied with other interests and therefore not focusing on food, or they did more exercise on holiday than at home.

2   A food journal can be done by a patient for 3–7 days to help detect dietary patterns and behaviors. Food journals include such details as time and place of meals and snacks eaten and description and quantity of food and beverages. Apart from gaining an insight into any possible behavioral problems, it also reduces reliance on memory and is a written learning tool. An advantage to food journals is that patients tend to become more aware of their own diet habits. Patients who record their daily intake tend to be more conscientious about food choices and portions than patients not keeping a journal. Food journals are also frequently used in treatment for obesity. As well as providing a record of reported food intake and eating behavior at baseline, the diet diary can be used throughout management to review and plan for future treatment. A diet diary encourages the patient to be actively involved in treatment and to take responsibility for making dietary and other behavior changes. It may also provide an indication of the patient's motivation, ways of improving motivation, and implementing change. It can also be very helpful to the patient to identify their own sabotaging factors.

The dietary history becomes the basis for discussion of eating habits. Any changes must be (as far as possible) acceptable to the patient in terms of palatability and practicality; otherwise, the patient will not adhere with the dietary advice. An understanding of the patient's lifestyle, including financial concerns, time constraints, and cultural issues, is also important. In addition to assessing the eating patterns of a patient, calculating an estimated amount of calories for weight loss may be helpful to set the stage for treatment. There are several predictive equations to estimate calorie needs. The most common equations used include the Harris–Benedict equation, the Mifflin–St Jeor method, and those of the IOM and the WHO.

Table 8.1 Equations used to predict patient's energy requirements.

Resting energy expenditure (REE) or resting metabolic rate (RMR) equations:
weight (WT) in kg; height (HT) in cm.

Harris–Benedict	Female: $655.1 + (9.6 \times WT) + (1.8 \times HT) - (4.7 \times age)$ Male: $66.5 + (13.8 \times WT) + (5.0 \times HT) - (6.8 \times age)$
Mifflin–St Jeor	Female: $(10 \times WT) + (6.25 \times HT) - (5 \times age) - 161$ Male: $(10 \times WT) + (6.25 \times HT) - (5 \times age) + 5$
WHO	Female: $(7.4 \times WT) + (482 \times HT) + 217$ Male: $(16.6 \times WT) + (77 \times HT) + 572$

Total energy expenditure (TEE) calculation

to estimate TEE, multiply REE by an activity factor:		Female	Male
Very light	Driving, typing, sewing, ironing, cooking	1.3	1.3
Light	Walking 3 miles/h, house cleaning, golf, child care	1.5	1.6
Moderate	Walking 4 miles/h, dancing, tennis, cycling	1.6	1.7
Heavy	Running, soccer, basketball, football	1.9	2.1

Total energy expenditure equation:

IOM	Female: $354 - 6.91 \times age + PA \times (9.36 \times WT + 726 \times HT)$ Male: $662 - 9.53 \times age + PA \times (15.91 \times WT + 539.6 \times HT)$

Physical activity (PA)		Female	Male
Sedentary	Basic living activities only	1.0	1.0
Less active	1.5–3 miles/day at 3 miles/h	1.12	1.11
Active	3–10 miles/day at 3 miles/h	1.27	1.25
Very active	10+ miles/day at 3 miles/h	1.45	1.48

These equations can give the patient's approximate caloric intake for weight maintenance (Table 8.1). Consuming 4200 kJ (1000 kcal) per day below the estimated requirement will normally produce a weight loss of 0.5–1.0 kg/week. Giving a specific calorie range to aim for is helpful for many patients.

Assessing eating patterns

One of the most important features learned from taking a diet history is the patient's eating pattern. Eating patterns involve the distribution of food, portion sizes, timing, and speed of eating. Often the daily ingestion of food is unbalanced and erratic. People will leave large time gaps between meals or skip meals altogether, leading to extreme hunger and food-seeking behavior. Mostly the food sought at this time is convenience food, which is easily accessible, gives instant gratification, and comes prepackaged. Convenience foods are mostly of low-satiety, high-energy, and high-fat value. When these foods are combined with increased hunger, the individual is predisposed to overconsumption, that is, eating beyond their energy requirements. If a meal is eaten at this time, often larger portions than normal are consumed in haste, with no adjustment to body satiety cues. Although the number of meals in a day might be low, the total energy intake is often high. Therefore, an energy deficit created by skipping a meal or lengthening the time between meals is not achieved.

Specific strategies to help patients reduce calories

Adopting healthier eating patterns

An initial goal is to help patients achieve a structured and planned eating schedule. It is best to eat regularly, leaving enough time to become hungry, but not ravenous, between meals. Eating slowly can help one to notice hunger and satiety cues earlier and ultimately leads to decreased consumption. Techniques to slow the pace of consumption include putting the cutlery down between bites, pausing during the meal, and chewing food well before swallowing. Other people may eat regularly but consume large portions. An energy deficit could be achieved by reducing the size or composition of the meals. For instance, less food fits on a salad plate compared to a dinner plate but the plate still looks full. Changing the type of food can be helpful; it is harder to overconsume bread that has many grains in it than it is to overconsume white bread, due to its texture and density. Assisting people in recognizing the feeling of satiety rather than being overly full and practicing stopping eating at the point of satisfaction, not fullness, is useful when aiming for portion control.

Partial meal replacement therapy

Partial meal replacement means that some of the daily meals (either one to two main meals and/or one to two snacks) are replaced with supplemented, portion-controlled food. Meal replacements are foods that are designed to take the place of a meal while at the same time providing nutrients and good taste within a fixed caloric limit. Examples include frozen entrees, canned beverages, and bars. Patients who use partial meal replacements lose on average 2.5 kg more than those consuming conventional food. Partial meal replacements appear to have advantages over full meal replacements as they offer participants choice and flexibility in social situations while reducing decision making at other times. Partial meal replacements are often successful in maintaining weight loss after an initial, intensive period of weight loss.

Reducing energy density

Energy density is based on the energy content per gram of food. The energy density of a food is thought to be low if it is less than 4 kJ/g (1 kcal/g), moderate if it is 4–6 kJ/g (1–1.5 kcal/g), and high if it is more than 6 kJ/g (more than 1.5 kcal/g). Energy density is related mostly to the water, fiber, and fat content of the food. Adding bulky, low-energy foods to the diet promotes satiety without adding unnecessary calories. Dry foods and high-fat foods such as pretzels, cheese, egg yolks, potato chips, and red meat have a high energy density. Diets containing low-energy-dense foods have been shown to control hunger and result in decreased caloric intake and weight loss. Soups and salads have been shown to be particularly helpful in reducing energy intake. Including soups and salads as pre-meals or as snacks and replacing soft drinks with water in the daily diet may assist in avoiding high-energy snacking and meals. The energy density of selected foods is shown in Figure 8.1.

Fixed-energy diets

A fixed-energy diet is one method of achieving an energy deficit. Intake is limited by controlling portion sizes, menu choice, and composition. These diets are often around 5 MJ (1200 kcal) for women and 7.5 MJ (1800 kcal) for men and are considered moderate hypocaloric diets. There is minimal

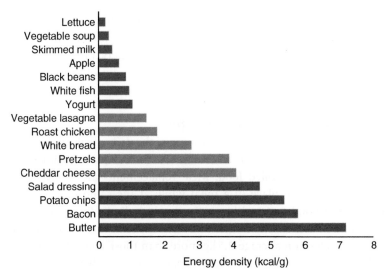

Figure 8.1 Energy density of selected foods.
Source: www.obesityonline.org.

self-monitoring, choice, or freedom. Lack of variety and departure from normal eating patterns often result in lack of compliance, although many people do find these diets helpful as they reduce decision making and, if followed accurately, are successful. There are many commercial programs that supply these diets, either in storefront offices, over the Internet, or by home delivery.

Very-low-energy (calorie) diets (VLED or VLCD)

Very-low-energy (calorie) diets (VLED or VLCD) provide approximately 3.4 MJ (approximately 800 kcal) per day and are lower than an individual's resting metabolic rate (RMR). These products contain the recommended dietary intake (RDI) for minerals and vitamins, electrolytes, and fatty acids and provide between 0.8 and 1.5 g of high-quality protein per kilogram of ideal body weight. VLED should only be used under medical supervision. The average weight loss for those who maintain the program is approximately 22 kg for women and 32 kg for men. Patients normally regain about 35–50% of their lost weight within 1 year; 10–20% regain all their weight and similar percentages apply to those who maintain their weight loss. Long-term results are generally no better (but no worse either) than other methods of weight loss. Improvement in the metabolic syndrome has been demonstrated using a VLED. Glycemic control improves within 1 week of starting the VLED, blood pressure can reduce by 8–13%, total serum cholesterol by 5–25%, and triglycerides by 15–50%. Reports of mood improvement may be attributed to accompanying behavior therapy programs, the weight loss seen, the feeling of control, or due to eating higher-quality food.

Low-carbohydrate or higher-protein diets

A low-carbohydrate diet contains less than 40% of total energy from carbohydrate. A higher-protein diet contains over 20% of total energy consumed as protein, and it is very high if the protein content is greater than 30% of the total energy. It is widely acknowledged that protein helps to suppress appetite more than fat or carbohydrate. This reduces the amount eaten at subsequent meals and also minimizes the likelihood of snacking. Some evidence suggests that a protein intake of 1.5 g/kg of bodyweight and less than 200 g of carbohydrate per day may increase thermogenesis and enhance glycemic control better than a diet that is low in protein and high in carbohydrate. High-protein, low-calorie diets are attractive as they induce ketogenesis and initially produce larger weight loss due to fluid depletion and the formation of ketones, which may help to suppress appetite. This in turn promotes reduced caloric intake. It remains controversial whether it is the calorie content or the macronutrient composition that is the major weight-loss-inducing factor in low-carbohydrate diets. Common adverse effects include fatigue (due to a depletion of glycogen), dizziness, headache or nausea (thought to be caused by sodium loss), constipation, halitosis, and muscle cramps, all of which occur more frequently in low-carbohydrate diets compared with conventional weight loss diets. Many low-carbohydrate diets restrict the intake of fruit, vegetables, and whole grains, which provide essential minerals and vitamins and are likely to prevent cancers. High-protein diets may also lead to increased calcium loss.

Ten practical dietary suggestions for most patients are listed in Box 8.2.

Box 8.2 Useful dietary behavioral strategies for patients wanting to lose weight.

1. Use a smaller plate

2. Do not skip meals

3. Do eat more of the day's calories earlier and fewer later if possible

4. Keep a food diary and annotate it with cues for "unhealthy eating," for example, emotions and circumstances that make this more likely

5. Eat slowly and stop when you are no longer hungry as opposed to when you feel overly full

6. Do not ingest calories in response to thirst, that is, drink water, not juice or soda

7. Avoid the feeling of starvation as you may overeat at the next opportunity

8. Do not go shopping for food while you are hungry

9. Do not keep tempting unhealthy foods or snacks in the house

10. Try to reduce the energy density of the foods you eat

Pitfalls
- Telling a patient what to eat to lose weight without first taking a diet history may lead to resistance and misdirection.
- Focusing on carbohydrates and fats in the diet instead of total calories may lead to less optimal weight loss.
- Using the patient's food diary as an accurate record of her caloric intake is misleading—patients under-report caloric intake.

Key web links

Dietary Guidelines for Americans, 2010. http://www.cnpp.usda.gov/publications/dietary guidelines/2010/policydoc/policydoc.pdf [accessed on December 29, 2012].
MyPlate. http://www.choosemyplate.gov/ [accessed on December 29, 2012].

American Medical Association. Assessment and management of adult obesity: A primer for physicians. *Dietary management.* http://www.ama-assn.org/ama/pub/physician-resources/public-health/general-resources-health-care-professionals/roadmaps-clinical-practice-series/assessment-management-adult-obesity.shtml [accessed on December 29, 2012].

Further reading

Foster, G.D., Wyatt, H.R., Hill, J.O. *et al.* (2010) Weight and metabolic outcomes after 2 years on a low-carbohydrate versus low-fat diet. A randomized trial. *Annals of Internal Medicine*, 153, 147–157.

Jebb, S., Ahern, A., Olson, A.D. *et al.* (2011) Primary care referral to a commercial provider for weight loss treatment versus standard care: A randomized controlled trial. *Lancet*, 378, 1485–1492.

Larsen, T.M., Dalskov, S.M., Baak, M.V. *et al.* (2010) Diets with high or low protein content and glycemic index for weight loss maintenance. *New England Journal of Medicine*, 363, 2102–2113.

Mozaffarian, D., Hao, T., Rimm, E.B., Willett, W.C. & Hu, F.B. (2011) Changes in diet and lifestyle and long-term weight gain in women and men. *New England Journal of Medicine*, 364, 2392–2404.

Rock, C.L., Flatt, S.W., Sherwood, N.E., Karanja, N., Pakiz, B. & Thomson, C.A. (2010) Effect of a free prepared meal and incentivized weight loss program on weight loss and weight loss maintenance in obese and overweight women. A randomized controlled trial. *Journal of American Medical Association*, 304, 1803–1811.

Sacks, F.M., Bray, G.A., Carey, V.J. *et al.* (2009) Comparison of weight-loss diets with different compositions of fat, protein, and carbohydrates. *New England Journal of Medicine*, 360, 859–873.

CHAPTER 9

Physical Activity and Exercise

Key points

- The primary benefits of exercise are to improve cardiorespiratory fitness, reduce obesity-related cardiovascular health risks, and preserve lean body mass.
- Whereas *physical activity* consists of any bodily movement that increases energy expenditure, for example, activities of daily living (ADLs), *exercise* is defined as planned, structured, and repetitive bodily movement done to improve or maintain one or more components of physical fitness. Weight loss counseling should encourage both entities.
- The physical activity prescription should specify the Frequency, Intensity, Timing, and Type of activity that can be safely Enjoyed and achieved by the patient. This is called the FITTE principle.
- People vary a great deal in how much physical activity is needed to achieve and maintain a healthy weight; however, 5 h or more of physical activity a week is recommended to lose weight and maintain weight loss.
- Most forms of physical activity have a lower contribution to net energy balance than many patients believe.

CASE STUDIES

Case study 1

JP is a 42-year-old male with a BMI of 32 kg/m². He is following a calorie-reduced diet and has lost 3 kg over the past 2 months. He is interested in starting an exercise program.

Comment: After taking a physical activity history, you learn that he enjoys walking and has no limitation to exercise. Using the FITTE principle, you devise a plan for him to walk 5 days a week (3 work days and 2 weekends) for 20–30 min at a pace of 4.0 miles/h. He will gauge the intensity by using the talk test. He will purchase a pedometer to track his steps with the goal of increasing them by 10% every week. A follow-up visit was set for 1 month to review progress.

Practical Manual of Clinical Obesity, First Edition. Robert Kushner, Victor Lawrence and Sudhesh Kumar.

> **Case study 2**
> KN is a 35-year-old female with an initial BMI of 36 kg/m². She has been following a
> calorie-reduced diet for 10 months and has successfully lost 11% of initial body weight.
> She has increased her ADLs and walks for 1 h 3 days a week with a friend. She is also
> thinking about starting a yoga class at her community center. KN is concerned about
> her ability to keep the weight off long term.
>
> **Comment**: You inform her that one of the most significant predictors of weight
> maintenance is high levels of physical activity. And although individuals vary, engaging
> in more than 250 min/week of moderate-intensity physical activity may be needed to be
> successful. Accordingly, you encourage her to increase her lifestyle activities, such as
> walking, and to begin an exercise and sport activity that she would find enjoyable, such
> as bicycling, jogging, or tennis.

Exercise and weight reduction

Physical activity and exercise is an important adjunct to dietary
restriction even though exercise alone is only moderately effective for
weight loss. Most studies show that exercise results in a weight loss of
between 1 and 3 kg greater than non-exercise control groups. This is to
be expected, since most exercise interventions aim to increase energy
expenditure by 1000–1500 kcal/week, whereas a caloric deficit of 500–
1000 kcal/day is usually induced by energy-restricted diets. In contrast,
the primary benefits of exercise are to improve cardiorespiratory fitness,
reduce obesity-related cardiovascular health risks (hypertension,
diabetes, dyslipidemia), preserve lean body mass, reduce total abdominal fat and visceral fat, and enhance a sense of well-being *independent* of
weight or BMI. Additionally, a high level of exercise appears to be one
of the most important factors in the maintenance of the weight lost. For
these reasons, physical activity counseling should be included in all
obesity care practices.

Exercise and obesity-related CVD

Insulin resistance and T2DM

Insulin resistance is an important feature in the development of glucose
intolerance and T2DM. An acute exercise bout increases postexercise
insulin sensitivity, an effect that is maintained for 48–72 h. Insulin sensitivity is increased in those skeletal muscles that have been active during
the exercise bout. Exercise training improves skeletal muscle insulin sensitivity of glucose transport in both insulin-sensitive and insulin-resistant
adults with obesity. Thus, regular exercise can reduce insulin resistance

and improve glucose tolerance in obesity and T2DM and reduce the risk of T2DM in high-risk populations, even in the absence of changes in weight and/or body composition.

Blood lipids

Exercise training has consistently been shown to increase HDL-cholesterol levels. Reductions in total cholesterol, LDL cholesterol, and triglycerides may also occur with training. Concurrent diet-induced weight loss potentiates the reductions in LDL cholesterol, total cholesterol, and triglycerides, and exercise training may attenuate HDL reduction with low-fat diets. In sedentary overweight or mildly obese subjects with dyslipidemia, regular exercise improves overall lipoprotein profile. High-amount/high-intensity exercise has significantly more beneficial effects on plasma lipoproteins than low-amount/high-intensity or low-amount/low-intensity exercise. The beneficial effects on HDL are sustained up to 2 weeks after exercise cessation, but the effects on VLDL and LDL appear to be relatively short lived. Aerobic exercise training has also been shown to reduce plasma triglyceride and tends to increase HDL cholesterol in obese or overweight children.

Blood pressure

Blood pressure changes associated with endurance exercise training show average systolic and diastolic blood pressure reductions of 3.0 and 2.4 mmHg, respectively. The reductions were more pronounced in hypertensive subjects (6.9 and 4.9 mmHg) than in the normotensive group (1.9 and 1.6 mmHg). No clear relationships between the blood pressure response and characteristics of the exercise programs (exercise intensity, duration, frequency) are seen. The blood-pressure-reducing effect of endurance exercise is independent of initial body mass and percent body fat or changes in body weight and composition. When comparing the effects of a combined intervention including dietary energy restriction and exercise training with the effect of diet alone, no additional reduction of blood pressure is found over that in exercise trials alone.

Physical activity and exercise counseling

There is a distinction between physical activity and exercise. Whereas *physical activity* consists of any bodily movement that increases energy expenditure, for example, ADLs like walking, climbing stairs, gardening, and so on, *exercise* is defined as planned, structured, and repetitive bodily movement done to improve or maintain one or more components of physical fitness. Weight loss counseling should encourage both entities as part of treatment.

It is important to ask patients what their current level of physical activity is and whether they engage in any exercise. Non-judgmental and informative questions include, "What is the most physically active thing you do on a daily basis?" "What types of physical activities do you enjoy?" and "Have you thought about increasing the amount of physical activity in which you participate?" Equal attention should be paid to barriers to physical activity, such as time restraints, lack of access to recreational or exercise facilities, low self-confidence, or poor conditioning. Understanding the patient's barriers to physical activity can help develop a personalized physical activity prescription.

Getting the patient started

Focusing on simple ways to add physical activity into the normal daily routine through leisure activities, travel, and domestic work should be suggested. Studies have demonstrated that lifestyle activities are as effective as structured exercise programs in improving cardiorespiratory fitness and weight loss. Examples include walking, using the stairs, doing home and yard work, and engaging in sport activities. Furthermore, the benefits from physical activity can be achieved by the accumulation of activity in shorter bouts, for example, brisk walking for 15 min twice daily. The physical activity prescription should specify the Frequency, Intensity, Timing, and Type of activity that can be safely Enjoyed and achieved by the patient. This is called the FITTE principle. An example would be to walk 5 times/week for 30 min at a pace of 3.8 miles/h (Table 9.1). Asking the patient to wear a pedometer to monitor total accumulation of steps as part of the ADLs is a useful strategy. Monitoring steps can motivate patients to increase time spent in physical activity and reduce inactivity.

Prescriptions of frequency and duration of exercise are simple and straightforward. The more difficult aspects of exercise prescription are defining and monitoring the intensity of exercise. The intensity of exercise can be prescribed as an absolute intensity (VO_2 or MET) or a

Table 9.1 An exercise prescription.

Type of exercise	Walking
Frequency	5 times/week
Intensity	3.8 miles/h or a 6–7 RPE
Timing	In the morning before work
Duration	45 min
Enjoyment	Walk with a partner

relative intensity, such as a percentage of the maximal oxygen uptake (% VO_2max) or maximal heart rate (%HRmax). One MET (metabolic equivalent) represents an individual's energy expenditure while sitting quietly (3.5 mL O_2/kg/min). MET values of selected activities and their classification as light-, moderate-, or vigorous-intensity activities are given in Table 9.2. Relative intensities can be classified as shown in Table 9.3. Since VO_2max is difficult to measure in non-laboratory exercise settings, prescription of exercise intensity is usually based on heart rate (as percentage of measured, but usually estimated, maximal heart rate (% HRmax)) or heart rate reserve (% HRR) (= maximal heart rate – resting heart rate) or, most commonly, on subjective feelings of exertion (RPE (rating of perceived exertion)). This is based on the linear relationship between % HRmax or % HRR and RPE, on one hand, and % VO_2max, on the other.

Currently there is no evidence that exercise intensity has an effect on weight reduction or weight maintenance independent of its contribution to total energy expenditure. However, more vigorous exercise will allow the individual to attain a preset energy expenditure in a shorter time. Two caveats are important: more vigorous exercise is associated with a higher injury risk, and it may lead to higher dropout rates from the program. A careful balance between time restraints and attainment of sufficiently high total energy expenditure therefore needs to be sought for each individual. The importance of improving aerobic fitness needs to be stressed because this will enable the obese individual to perform a higher workload with less physical stress.

Setting goals

There is no precise goal regarding the amount of physical activity needed for losing weight and maintaining weight loss. However, the American College of Sports Medicine (ACSM) recommends that overweight and obese individuals progressively increase to a minimum of 150 min of moderate-intensity physical activity per week as a first goal. For long-term weight loss, higher amounts of exercise (e.g., 200–300 min/week or ≥2000 kcal/week) are needed. The Dietary Guidelines for Americans 2005 found compelling evidence that at least 60–90 min of daily moderate-intensity physical activity (7–10.5 h/week) is needed to sustain weight loss. The ACSM also recommends that resistance exercise supplement the endurance exercise program. These recommendations will feel daunting to most patients and need to be implemented gradually. It is useful to remind them that lesser levels of physical activity are beneficial for long-term health. Many patients would benefit from consultation with an exercise physiologist or personal trainer. Figure 9.1 depicts a physical activity recommendation pathway for clinical counseling.

Table 9.2 Energy cost of various physical activities expressed as METs (ratio of work metabolic rate to resting metabolic rate)

Light <3.0 METs	Moderate 3.0–6.0 METs	Vigorous >6.0 METs
Walking, jogging and running	*Walking, jogging and running*	*Walking, jogging and running*
Walking slowly around home, store or office = 2.0[a]	Walking 3.0 mph (4.8 km/h) = 3.3[a]	Walking at very very brisk pace (4.5 mph, 7.2 km/h) = 6.3[a]
	Walking at very brisk pace (4 mph, 6.4 km/h) = 5.0[a]	Walking/hiking at moderate pace and grade with no or light pack (<10 lb, 4.5 kg) = 7.0 Hiking at steep grades and pack 10–42 lb, 4.5–19 kg = 7.5–9.0 Jogging at 5 mph (8 km/h) = 8.0[a] Jogging at 6 mph (9.7 km/h) = 10.0[a] Running at 7 mph (11.3 km/h) = 11.5[a]
Household and occupation	*Household and occupation*	*Household and occupation*
Sitting—using computer, work at desk using light hand tools = 1.5	Cleaning—heavy: washing windows, car, clean garage = 3.0	Shoveling sand, coa, etc. = 7.0
Standing, performing light work such as making bed, washing dishes, ironing, preparing food, or store clerk = 2.0–2.5	Sweeping floors or carpet, vacuuming, mopping = 3.0–3.5	Carrying heavy loads such as bricks = 7.5
	Carpentry—general = 3.6	Heavy farming such as bailing hay = 8.0
	Carrying & stacking wood = 5.5 Mowing lawn—walk power mower = 5.5	Shoveling, digging ditches = 8.5
Leisure time and sports	*Leisure time and sports*	*Leisure time and sports*
Arts & crafts, playing cards = 1.5	Badminton—recreational = 4.5	Basketball game = 8.0
Billiards = 2.5	Basketball—shooting around = 4.5	Bicycling—on flat: moderate effort (12–14 mph, 18–21 km/h) = 8.0

Table 9.2 (cont'd)

Light <3.0 METs	Moderate 3.0–6.0 METs	Vigorous >6.0 METs
Boating—power = 2.5	Bicycling—on flat: light effort (10–12 mph, 15–18 km/h) = 6.0	
Croquet = 2.5		Bicycling—fast (14–16 mph, 21–24 km/h) = 10
Darts = 2.5	Dancing—ballroom, slow = 3.0	Skiing cross country—slow (2.5 mph, 3.8 km/h) = 7.0
Fishing—sitting = 2.5	Dancing—ballroom, fast = 4.5	
Playing (most) musical intruments = 2.0–2.5	Fishing from river bank and walking = 4.0	Skiing cross country—fast (5.0–7.9 mph, 7.5–12 km/h) = 9.0
	Golf—walking pulling clubs = 4.3	
	Sailing boat, wind surfing = 3.0	Soccer—casual = 7.0
	Swimming leisurely = 6.0[b]	Soccer—competitive = 10.0
	Table tennis = 4.0	Swimming—moderate/hard = 8–11[b]
	Tennis doubles = 5.0	Tennis singles = 8.0
	Volleyball—noncompetitive = 3.0–4.0	Volleyball—competitive at gym or beach = 8.0

[a]Adapted from Haskell, W.L. et al. (2007) Medicine and Science in Sports and Exercise, 39, 1423–1434, with permission from Lippincott Williams & Wilkins.
[b]On flat, hard surface.
MET values can vary substantially from person to person during swimming as a result of different strokes and skill levels.

Table 9.3 Classification of relative intensity of exercise based on 20–60 minutes of endurance training

% HRmax	% VO$_2$ max or % HRR	RPE	Intensity classification
<35	<30	<10	Very light
35–59	30–49	10–11	Light
60–79	50–74	12–13	Moderate (somewhat hard)
80–89	75–84	14–16	Heavy
≥90	≥85	>16	Very heavy

Adapted from American College of Sports Medicine (1990) Medicine and Science in Sports and 22, 265–274, with permission from Lippincott Williams & Wilkins.
VO$_2$max, maximal oxygen uptake; HRR, heart rate reserve (maximal heart rate – resting heart rate); HRmax, maximal heart rate; RPE, rating of perceived exertion (20-point Borg scale).

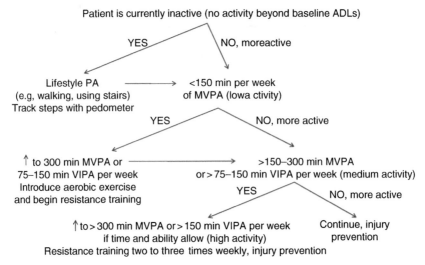

Figure 9.1 Physical activity (PA) recommendations for obesity based on activity level assessment. MVPA = moderately vigorous physical activity = 3.0–5.9 times the amount of energy expended at rest. VIPA = vigorous-intensity physical activity = ≥6.0 times the amount of energy expended at rest. Adapted from American College of Sports Medicine [1], with permission from Lippincott Williams & Wilkins.

Pitfalls
- Exercise alone rarely leads to significant weight loss—it must be accompanied by dietary restriction.
- Counseling will not be successful unless the challenges and obstacles to increasing physical activity are directly addressed.
- The goal to accumulate 5 h or more per week of moderate-intensity physical activity is daunting! Start slow and progress on a weekly basis.
- Patients will not consistently engage in physical activity and exercise unless it fits their lifestyle.

Key web links

2008 Physical Activity Guidelines for Americans. http://www.health.gov/paguidelines [accessed on December 29, 2012].

Dietary Guidelines for Americans 2005. http://www.health.gov/dietaryguidelines/ [accessed on December 29, 2012].

Physical activity management. In: *Assessment and Management of Adult Obesity: A Primer for Physicians.* http://www.ama-assn.org/ama1/pub/upload/mm/433/booklet2.pdf [accessed on December 29, 2012].

Reference

1 American College of Sports Medicine. (2009) Appropriate physical activity intervention strategies for weight loss and prevention of weight regain for adults. *Medicine & Science in Sports & Exercise*, 41, 459–471. http://www.acsm-msse.org/ [accessed on December 29, 2012].

Further reading

American College of Sports Medicine. (2011) Quantity and quality of exercise for and maintaining cardiorespiratory, musculoskeletal, and neuromotor fitness in apparently healthy adults: Guidance for prescribing exercise. *Medicine & Science in Sports & Exercise*, 43, 1334–1359.

Bassett, D.R., Wyatt, H.R., Thompson, H., Peters, J.C. & Hill, J.O. (2010) Pedometer-measured physical activity and health behaviors in U.S. adults. *Medicine & Science in Sports & Exercise*, 42, 1819–1825.

Church, T.S., Martin, C.K., Thompson, A.M., Earnest, C.P., Mikus, C.R. & Blair, S.N. (2009) Changes in weight, waist circumference and compensatory responses with different doses of exercise among sedentary, overweight postmenopausal women. *PLoS One*, 4, 1–11.

Gordon-Larson, P., Hou, N., Sidney, S. *et al.* (2009) Fifteen-year longitudinal trends in walking patterns and their impact on weight change. *American Journal of Clinical Nutrition*, 89, 19–26.

Jakicic, J.M., Marcus, B.H., Lang, W. & Janney, C. (2008) Effect of exercise on 24-month weight loss maintenance in overweight women. *Archives of Internal Medicine*, 168, 1550–1559.

Jonas, S. & Phillips, E.M. (eds) (2009) *ACSM's Exercise is Medicine: A Clinicians Guide to Exercise Prescription*. Lippincott, Williams & Wilkins, Philadelphia.

Kokkinos, P. & Myers, J. (2010) Exercise and physical activity. Clinical outcomes and applications. Circulation, 122, 1637–1648.

O'Donovan, G., Blazevich, A.J., Boreham, C. *et al.* (2010) The ABC of physical activity for health: A consensus statement from the British Association of Sports and Exercise Sciences. *Journal of Sports Sciences*, 28, 573–591.

Schwartz, A. & Doucet, D. (2010) Relative changes in resting energy expenditure during weight loss: A systematic review. *Obesity Reviews*, 11, 531–547.

CHAPTER 10

Behavior Therapy

Key points

- The goal of behavioral treatment is to help patients with obesity identify and modify their eating and activity habits by providing them with a set of principles, skills, and techniques.
- Behavior therapy provides a goal-oriented approach to weight loss.
- Self-monitoring (diet, physical activity, body weight) is the most important component of behavioral treatment for obesity.
- Motivational interviewing (MI) is a client-centered, directive method for enhancing intrinsic motivation to change by exploring and resolving ambivalence.

CASE STUDIES

Case study 1

SA is a 38-year-old female with a BMI of 34.5 kg/m². Due to increasing blood pressure and development of GERD, you advise her to lose weight. She is interested but does not know how to start since she has never been in a weight management program.

Comment: To begin, you ask her to begin tracking her diet, noting time, place, and amount of food and beverage consumed along with identifying any triggers for emotional eating. You also ask her to purchase a pedometer to track her daily steps. With her input, you mutually develop short-term goals for her to achieve that include reducing total calories to 1400 kcal/day, not skipping breakfast, planning her diet in advance, adding a serving of fruit and vegetables with each meal, and accumulating 30 min of moderately vigorous intensity physical activity on most days of the week. You set up a follow-up visit in 1 month to review progress.

Case study 2

LK is a 45-year-old female with a BMI of 29.8 kg/m² who presents with a weight gain of 9 kg over the past 3 years. She has a long history of anxiety and emotional eating. Since her oldest child left for college, she has turned to food for comfort. She has always put

---

Practical Manual of Clinical Obesity, First Edition. Robert Kushner, Victor Lawrence and Sudhesh Kumar.
© 2013 John Wiley & Sons, Ltd. Published 2013 by John Wiley & Sons, Ltd.

others before herself and is having difficulty motivating herself to eat healthier and get more exercise. LK has a good fund of knowledge regarding diet but cannot seem to make the right choices.

Comment: To focus on emotional eating, you ask her to keep a "food and mood diary" where she records the antecedents (how she feels before eating) and consequences (how she feels after eating) in addition to the type and amount of food/beverage consumed. By better knowing her trigger situations and emotions, she can begin to take control of her eating, develop a positive action plan, and adopt non-eating coping strategies.

Case study 3

MS is a 52-year-old male with a BMI of 38 kg/m² having medical problems significant for hypertension, T2DM, and mixed hyperlipidemia. He states that he wants to lose weight but is not motivated to change his diet or exercise.

Comment: Using the principles of MI, you express that losing weight can be challenging and behavior change is hard for many people. You ask him to reflect on the importance of his personal goal of reducing his medications and feeling better versus continuing his current diet and inactivity patterns. You encourage him to explore the barriers that make it difficult for him to make the small changes in diet and activity that are needed to reduce body weight. You actively listen and build his confidence in any changes that he feels he can implement over the coming weeks. A short-term goal is mutually agreed upon.

Principles of behavior therapy

The goal of behavioral treatment is to help patients with obesity identify and modify their eating and physical activity habits by providing them with a set of principles, skills, and techniques. Knowing what to do and how to be healthier is not intuitive for all patients. Behavior change is hard. Behavioral treatment is defined by the following three characteristics: (1) it specifies very clear goals in terms that can be easily measured; (2) treatment is process oriented, that is, focuses on the behaviors that trigger eating; and (3) it advocates small rather than large change. Behavior therapy teaches patients the process of evaluating antecedent events and consequences of problem behaviors. Such analysis highlights cues that are frequently associated with problem eating and activity behaviors (i.e., times, places, people), thus identifying opportunities for intervention. Problem behaviors are often triggered by a series of events that are linked together in a chain, as illustrated in Figure 10.1. Mapping the links in a behavioral chain can identify the source of the problem and suggest options for intervention. Patients are benefited from implementing a specific plan of action with defined and measurable goals.

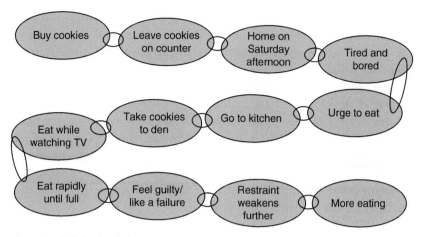

Figure 10.1 Behavioral chain.

Components of behavioral treatment

Behavior therapy provides a goal-oriented approach to weight loss. Patients are encouraged to set concrete, tangible goals with measurable outcomes. They should leave each visit with a strategy for how they will achieve their goals. This includes devising a detailed plan of what they will do, when and where they will do it, and how often. For example, helping patients develop a plan to walk around the neighborhood for 15 min on Monday, Wednesday, Thursday, and Saturday evenings, immediately after dinner, is more helpful than simply telling them to increase their physical activity. Patients should set small goals that they can attain in order to maximize feelings of success (which will reinforce their behavior). Small successes build upon each other until patients reach their ultimate goals. Behavioral treatment includes multiple components such as self-monitoring, stimulus control, diet, exercise, cognitive restructuring, social support, problem solving, and relapse prevention. This chapter highlights three of these components: self-monitoring, stimulus control, and cognitive restructuring. It then discusses the principles of MI.

Self-monitoring

Self-monitoring is probably the most important component of behavioral treatment for obesity. Patients keep detailed records of their food intake, physical activity, and weight throughout the treatment. They initially record the type, amount, and caloric value of foods eaten. This information is used to help patients reduce their caloric intake by 500–1000 kcal/day. As treatment progresses, patients may expand their self-monitoring to include additional data about times, places, and feelings associated with eating. This additional information typically reveals patterns of which patients may not be aware. For example, an individual may notice that he snacks excessively in the evenings. Another may realize that she often makes poor food choices when upset. Once problem areas have been identified, patient and practitioner work together to develop a plan to tackle the problem behavior. Individuals who regularly keep food records lose significantly more weight than those who record inconsistently. Self-recording can be completed on paper or electronically on the Internet or smart phone using any of the commercial tracking tools available. Regardless of the format used, it is important for the health-care provider to review the record with the patient as part of the counseling program.

Stimulus control

Stimulus control techniques help patients manage cues associated with eating and exercise behaviors. An event can become a cue to eat when it is repeatedly paired with eating. For example, walking into the kitchen often elicits a desire to eat because this room is so strongly associated with food. People rarely experience a food craving when in the attic or bathroom because of the absence of cues in these areas. Many events can prompt a desire to eat. The most obvious are the sight and smell of food. There is truth in the old adage "out of sight, out of mind." Behavior therapy teaches patients to reduce cues to unwanted eating by limiting exposure to problem foods. Patients are also taught to tackle cues related to time, place, and events with strategies such as: (1) limiting the places they eat (at home) to the kitchen or dining room, (2) eating at regular times of the day, and (3) refraining from engaging in other activities while eating (such as driving or watching television).

Stimulus control techniques can also target cues to promote healthy eating and activity habits. A patient might, for example, replace a cookie jar on the kitchen counter with a fruit basket. Another might place his walking shoes by the front door in order to prompt him to exercise. Behavioral treatment aims to decrease negative cues while increasing positive ones.

Cognitive restructuring

Negative thoughts can create obstacles to behavior change. A person who thinks, "I've blown my diet. I should just give up," after overeating is likely to respond differently from a person who thinks, "I know that wasn't the best choice I could have made, but I am going to stick with my plan for the rest of the day." The catastrophic thinking expressed by the first person is common among individuals attempting to lose weight and can lead patients to abandon their weight control efforts. Cognitive restructuring teaches patients to monitor maladaptive thoughts that may undermine their weight loss efforts and to replace them with more adaptive thoughts. Rational responses such as "Just because I ate an extra 300 cal tonight doesn'tmean I won'tbe able to lose weight" are more likely to elicit positive eating and activity habits. Cognitive restructuring is helpful in teaching patients to view a setback as a temporary lapse. The ultimate goal is to determine how lapses occurred and to develop strategies to prevent them. Cognitive techniques also can be used to help patients address body image concerns.

Motivational interviewing (MI)

Motivational interviewing (MI) is a client-centered, directive method for enhancing intrinsic motivation to change by exploring and resolving ambivalence. It focuses on what the patient wants and how the patient thinks and feels. According to MI, motivation to change is viewed as something that is evoked in the patient rather than imposed. It is the patient's task (not the clinician's) to articulate and resolve his or her own ambivalence. Intrinsic to this model is the concept that most patients are ambivalent about changing long-standing lifestyle behaviors, fearing that change will be difficult, uncomfortable, or depriving. The result of initiating a change plan when the patient is not ready often leads to frustration and disappointment. Patients frequently misattribute their lack of success to either a failure of effort (low willpower) or a poorly conceived diet. Patients who are ready and have thought about the benefits and difficulties of weight management are more likely to succeed. One helpful, simple, and rapid method to begin a readiness assessment is to "anchor" the patient's interest (or importance) and confidence to change on a numerical scale (Figure 10.2).

MI uses four general principles to explore and resolve ambivalence:
- *Express empathy*. Empathy refers to understanding the patient's feelings and perspectives without judging, criticizing, or blaming.
- *Develop discrepancy*. Create and amplify the discrepancy between present behavior and the patient's broader goals and values. Discrepancy has to do with the importance of change and the distance that the patient's behavior would need to travel in order to reach the desired level. This is called the "behavioral gap." The general approach is one that results in the patient reflecting on the actions and reasons for change.
- *Roll with resistance*. Although reluctance to change is to be expected in weight control, resistance (denial, arguing, putting up objections, yes–but statements) arises from the interpersonal interaction between the clinician and the patient. In this case, the therapeutic relationship is endangered and the counseling process becomes dysfunctional. It is a signal that the patient–clinician rapport is damaged. If this occurs, the

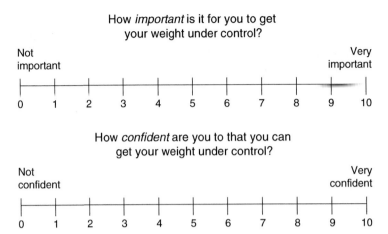

Figure 10.2 Numerical scales to assess patient's ambivalence.

clinician's task is to double back, understand the reason for resistance behavior, and redirect counseling. Rolling with resistance means not to confront the patient but allow them to express themselves. Using a reflective response serves to acknowledge the person's feelings or perceptions.

• *Support self-efficacy*. Self-efficacy refers to a person's belief in his or her ability to carry out and succeed with a specific task. Other common terms are hope and faith. A general goal of MI is to enhance the patient's confidence in her capacity to cope with obstacles and to succeed in change. The confidence scale used in Figure 10.2 quickly assesses the patient's level of confidence for a particular behavior change.

Pitfalls

• Assuming that patients will follow your behavioral advice without any ambivalence is mistaken. Change is hard.
• Assuming that patients intuitively know how to implement healthier behavior is incorrect. Behavior change is based on a set of skills.
• Assuming that giving patients general advice to lose weight, eat healthier, and get more exercise will be successful is misguided. Counseling should include goal setting.

Key web links

Communication and Counseling Strategies. In: *Assessment and Management of Adult Obesity: A Primer for Physicians*. American Medical Association Roadmaps for Clinical Practice, AMA, 2003. http://www.ama-assn.org/ama1/pub/upload/mm/433/booklet8.pdf [accessed on December 29, 2012].
http://www.motivationalinterview.org/index.html [accessed on December 29, 2012].

Further reading

Burke, L.E., Wang, J. & Sevick, M.A. (2011) Self-monitoring in weight loss: A systematic review of the literature. *Journal of the American Dietetic Association*, 111, 92–102.

Fabricatore, A.N. (2007) Behavior therapy and cognitive-behavioral therapy of obesity: Is there a difference? *Journal of the American Dietetic Association*, 107, 92–99.

Miller, W.R. & Rollnick, S. (eds) (2002) *Motivational Interviewing. Preparing People for Change*, 2nd edn. Guilford Press Publication, New York.

Rao, G., Burke, L.E., Spring, B.J. *et al.* (2011) New and emerging weight management strategies for busy ambulatory settings. A scientific statement from the American Heart Association. *Circulation*, 124, 1182–1203.

Rollnick, S., Butler, C.C., Kinnersley, P., Gregory, J. & Mash, B. (2010) Motivational interviewing. *BMJ*, 340, 1242–1245.

Watson, D.L. & Tharp, R.G. (eds) (2002) *Self-Directed Behavior*, 8th edn. Wadsworth Thompson Learning Publication, Belmont.

CHAPTER 11

Pharmacotherapy

Key points

- Adjuvant pharmacologic treatments should be considered for patients with a BMI over 30 kg/m^2 or with a BMI over 27 kg/m^2 who have concomitant obesity-related diseases.
- Phentermine and other sympathomimetic drugs are modestly effective in reducing hunger.
- Orlistat is a selective inhibitor of pancreatic lipase that reduces the intestinal digestion of fat. Mean weight loss (compared to placebo) is 2.51 kg at 6 months and 2.75 kg at 12 months.
- Two new medications, lorcaserin and combined phentermine/topiramate extended-release (ER), are available for adjunctive therapy.
- Pharmacotherapy should be considered only if the patient will be taking the medication in conjunction with an overall weight management program, including a reduced calorie diet and increased physical activity, and has realistic expectations of medication therapy.
- When possible, weight-gaining medications should be discontinued and replaced with weight-losing or weight-neutral medications.

CASE STUDIES

Case study 1

SK is a 44-year-old female with a BMI of 34 kg/m^2 and waist circumference of 90 cm. She has been weight cycling over the past two decades since she had pregnancies at ages 22, 24, and 27. SK has joined several commercial weight management programs, losing about 8% of her body weight each time followed by weight regain. She is knowledgeable about calories and portion sizes but finds it hard to stick to the meal plans. She was just diagnosed with pre-diabetes and is concerned about her inability to control her weight.

Comment: After counseling her on a healthy diet and physical activity plan, you review the role of adjunctive medications and prescribe orlistat 120 mg t.i.d. with meals. A follow-up visit is scheduled for 6 weeks.

Practical Manual of Clinical Obesity, First Edition. Robert Kushner, Victor Lawrence and Sudhesh Kumar.
© 2013 John Wiley & Sons, Ltd. Published 2013 by John Wiley & Sons, Ltd.

Case study 2

DM is a 32-year-old male with a BMI of 29.5 kg/m² and waist circumference of 95 cm. He was in good health until 2 years ago when he developed symptoms of a major depressive disorder (MDD). He has been seeing a clinical psychologist on a weekly basis and was prescribed mirtazapine 30 mg q.i.d for the depression and to improve sleep. Over this time, he has gained 20 lb despite trying to eat healthier and be more physically active. His MDD is improved but he is now concerned about increasing body weight.

Comment: After discussion with his psychiatrist, a decision was made to discontinue mirtazapine, a known weight-gaining medication, with a weight-neutral anti-depressant, bupropion.

Adjuvant pharmacologic treatments should be considered for patients with a BMI over 30 kg/m² or with a BMI over 27 kg/m² who also have concomitant obesity-related diseases and for whom dietary and physical activity therapy has not been successful. When prescribing an anti-obesity medication, patients should be actively engaged in a lifestyle program that provides the strategies and skills needed to effectively use the drug, since this support increases total weight loss.

There are several potential targets of pharmacologic therapy for obesity. The most thoroughly explored treatment is suppression of appetite via centrally active medications that alter monoamine neurotransmitters. A second strategy is to reduce the absorption of selective macronutrients from the GI tract, such as fat. These two mechanisms form the basis for currently prescribed anti-obesity agents.

The legacy of anti-obesity medications

In the past, anti-obesity drugs have been marred with concerns over safety and inappropriate usage, leading to several instances of market withdrawal due to serious adverse events. In 1997, fenfluramine and dexfenfluramine were withdrawn from the world market due to the development of cardiac valvular abnormalities and pulmonary hypertension. In the USA, the over-the-counter anorexiant phenylpropanolamine (PPA) was withdrawn in 2000 due to an independent risk for hemorrhagic stroke in women. The same year, the European Medicines Agency (EMEA) recommended withdrawal of several amphetamine derivative weight loss drugs from the market, including phentermine, diethylpropion, and mazindol. Rimonabant, a cannabinoid-1 receptor blocker, was approved by the EMEA in 2006 as an adjunct to diet and exercise for the treatment of obese or overweight patients with associated risk factors. However, the company withdrew its application to the US Food and Drug Administration (FDA) in June 2007 due to psychiatric safety considerations of depressed mood disorders and suicidal ideation. The EMEA subsequently withdrew rimonabant from all countries of the European Union in January 2009. Finally, sibutramine, an NE serotonin re-uptake inhibitor, was removed from the world market in 2010 for cardiovascular risk concerns after release of results from the Sibutramine Cardiovascular Outcomes Trial (SCOUT). Based on this controversial history, it is reasonable to assume that many physicians will be cautious when considering to prescribe a pharmacologic agent for obesity treatment. Similar to other medications used for chronic illness care, balancing risk with benefit is of paramount importance. It is important for physicians to educate themselves about new drugs regarding use, indications, outcomes, and side effects.

Drugs that reduce food intake primarily by acting on the CNS

Phentermine and other sympathomimetic drugs

The sympathomimetic drugs, benzphetamine, diethylpropion, phendimetrazine, and phentermine, are grouped together because they act like NE. Drugs in this group work by a variety of mechanisms, including the blockade of NE re-uptake from synaptic granules. All of these drugs are absorbed orally and reach peak blood concentrations within a short period. Side effects include dry mouth, constipation, and insomnia. Food intake is suppressed either by delaying the onset of a meal or by producing early satiety. One of the longest clinical trials of drugs in this group lasted 36 weeks and compared placebo treatment with continuous phentermine or intermittent phentermine. Both continuous and intermittent phentermine therapy produced more weight loss than placebo. In the drug-free periods, the patients treated intermittently slowed their weight loss, only to lose weight more rapidly when the drug was reinstituted. Phentermine and diethylpropion are classified by the US Drug Enforcement Administration as schedule IV drugs; benzphetamine and phendimetrazine are schedule III drugs. This regulatory classification indicates the US government's belief that they have the potential for abuse, although this potential appears to be very low. Phentermine and diethylpropion are approved for only a "few weeks," which is usually interpreted as up to 12 weeks. Weight loss with phentermine and diethylpropion persists for the duration of treatment, suggesting that tolerance does not develop to these drugs. If tolerance were to develop, the drugs would be expected to lose their effectiveness, and patients would require increased amounts of the drug to maintain weight loss. This does not occur.

Safety

The side-effect profiles for sympathomimetic drugs are similar. These agents produce insomnia, dry mouth, asthenia, and constipation. The safety of older sympathomimetic appetite-suppressant drugs has been the subject of considerable controversy because dextroamphetamine is addictive. The sympathomimetic drugs phentermine, diethylpropion, benzphetamine, and phendimetrazine have very little abuse potential, as assessed by the low rate of reinforcement when the drugs are self-injected intravenously by test animals. Sympathomimetic drugs can also increase blood pressure levels.

Phentermine and topiramate ER (Qsymia™, manufactured by Vivus, Inc.)

Phentermine and topiramate ER combines a catecholamine releaser and an anticonvulsant, respectively. Topiramate is currently approved by the US FDA as an anticonvulsant for the treatment of epilepsy and for the prophylaxis of migraine headaches. Weight loss was seen as an unintended side effect during clinical trials for epilepsy. The mechanism responsible for weight loss is uncertain but thought to be mediated through the modulation of gamma-aminobutyric acid (GABA) receptors, inhibition of carbonic anhydrase, and antagonism of glutamate to reduce food intake. Topiramate has been demonstrated to produce significant weight loss as a single agent in double-blind, placebo-controlled trials among obese subjects; however, the side effects of cognitive impairment and paresthesia limited its further research as a weight loss drug. The manufacturer's approach to improving the tolerability of topiramate was to combine a mild anorectic stimulant, phentermine, with a lower dose of topiramate ER. In two phase-III trials called EQUIP and CONQUER, both 1-year, randomized, placebo-controlled, double-blind clinical trials, three different strengths of a once-a-day formulation were tested: full strength dose (15 mg of phentermine and 92 mg of topiramate ER), mid-dose (7.5 mg of phentermine and 92 mg of topiramate ER), and low dose (3.75 mg of phentermine and 23 mg of topiramate ER). A description of the subject populations and weight loss outcomes is shown in Table 11.1. Subjects randomized to the full strength dose in the EQUIP and CONQUER trials lost an average of 10.9% and 9.8% body weight in 1 year (intention-to-treat (ITT) analysis) compared to 1.6% and 1.2% loss for placebo subjects, respectively. Significant improvements in fasting glucose, insulin, glycated hemoglobin, and lipid profile were also seen.

Dosing

Due to the dose-dependent side effects of the medication, an initial dose of 3.75/23 mg is prescribed daily for the first 14 days and then increased to 7.5/46 mg daily. Patients should be re-evaluated after 3 months; if 3% weight loss is not achieved by that time, either discontinue or escalate the dose to 15/92 mg for another 12 weeks. The next landmark time is at 6 months; discontinue the medication if the patient has not achieved at least 5% weight

Table 11.1 Comparison of the three medications that have submitted a new drug application (NDA) for FDA approval based on completion of 1-year phase-III trial data.

Drug	Number	BMI (mean, kg/m^2)	Age (mean, year)	mean percent wt loss (ITT)	Loss of >5% wt (%)	Loss of >10% wt (%)
Lorcaserin						
Placebo	1046	36.2	44.0	2.2	20.3	7.7
Lorcaserin	1081	36.2	43.8	5.8	47.5	22.6
Contrave[a]						
Placebo	581	36.2	43.7	1.3	16	7.0
N16/B360	578	36.2	44.4	5.0	39	20
N32/B360	583	36.1	44.4	6.1	48	25
Qsymia[b]						
Placebo	994	36.7	51.2	1.2	20.8	9.7
PHEN7.5/TPM46	498	36.2	51.1	7.8	62.1	49.1
PHEN15/TPM92	995	36.6	51.0	9.8	70.0	64.3

[a] Contrave is a fixed combination of naltrexone (N) and bupropion (B). Study drug contains either N 16 mg + B 360 mg or N 32 mg + B 360 mg.
[b] Qsymia is a fixed combination of phentermine (PHEN) and topiramate (TPM) ER. Study drug contains either PHEN 7.5 mg + TPM 46 mg or PHEN 15 mg + TPM 92 mg. Data presented are from OB 303 study.

loss. These 3- and 6-month weight loss cut points are included to optimize the risk–benefit ratio among patients who are deemed "non-responders."

Safety

The side effects of Qsymia™ (approved for use by US FDA) are due to both medications. The most commonly reported side effects resulting from phentermine are dry mouth and constipation. Side effects from topiramate are paresthesia, dysgeusia (abnormal taste), and disturbance in attention (cognitive impairment). The most significant concern of topiramate is an increased risk of orofacial clefts in infants exposed to the drug during the first trimester of pregnancy, a risk factor that is shared by all antiepileptic medications. Due to this concern, all women of childbearing age are required to be counseled on birth control at the initial and follow-up visits and have a pregnancy test before starting Qsymia and monthly thereafter during therapy.

Lorcaserin (Belviq™, manufactured by Arena Pharmaceuticals, Inc.)

Lorcaserin is a 5-HT2C receptor agonist. Previous experience with fenfluramine and dexfenfluramine demonstrated the anorexiant properties of activating the serotonergic system, particularly 5-HT2C receptors. However, the unintentional development of valvulopathy by interaction with several proteins found in heart valves, including 5-HT1B, 5-HT2A, and 5-HT2B receptors, mandated the identification of compounds selective for 5-HT2C receptors and free of valvular heart disease. Unlike the 5-HT2A and 5-HT2B receptors, there is little evidence for expression of 5-HT2C receptors outside of the CNS. Lorcaserin is a full agonist at the 5-HT2C receptor with a potency of approximately 10 nM and approximately 15- and 100-fold selectivity over the 5-HT2A and 5-HT2B receptors, respectively. In two phase-III trials called BLOOM and BLOSSOM, both randomized, placebo-controlled, double-blind clinical trials, subjects randomized to lorcaserin 10 mg twice daily lost an average of 5.8% of body weight in 1 year (ITT analysis) compared to 2.2% for placebo subjects, respectively. Significant improvements in fasting glucose, insulin, and lipid profile were also seen. Echocardiographic valvulopathy occurred in 2% of subjects on placebo and lorcaserin 10 mg b.i.d. (no significant difference).

Dosing

The dose for Belviq™ (approved for use by US FDA) is one tablet of 10 mg twice daily. Clinicians are instructed to discontinue the medication if 5% weight loss is not achieved by 3 months of therapy. The 3-month weight loss cut point is included to optimize the risk–benefit ratio among patients who are deemed "non-responders."

Safety

The most common side effects of lorcaserin (occurring in greater than 5% of patients) are headache, dizziness, fatigue, nausea, dry mouth, and constipation.

Drugs that reduce fat absorption

Orlistat: pharmacology and efficacy

Orlistat is a potent and selective inhibitor of pancreatic lipase that reduces the intestinal digestion of fat. The drug has a dose-dependent effect on fecal fat loss, increasing it to approximately 30% on a diet that has 30% of its energy as fat. Orlistat has lesser or little effect on subjects eating a low-fat diet, as might be anticipated from its mechanism of action. A number of long-term clinical trials (1–4 years) with orlistat have been published. In one trial, by the end of year 1, the placebo-treated patients lost 6.1% of their initial body weight and the drug-treated patients lost 10.2%. In a second 2-year study, at the end of year 1, the weight loss was −8.7 kg in the orlistat-treated group and −5.8 kg in the placebo group ($P<0.001$). During the second year, those switched to placebo after year 1 reached the same weight as those treated with placebo for 2 years (−4.5% in those with placebo for 2 years and −4.2% in those switched to placebo during year 2).

A 4-year double-blind, randomized, placebo-controlled trial with orlistat (XENDOS) treated a total of 3304 overweight patients, 21% of whom had impaired glucose tolerance. The lowest body weight was achieved during the first year and was more than 11% below baseline in the orlistat-treated group and 6% below baseline in the placebo-treated group. Over the remaining 3 years of the trial, there was a small regain in weight, such that, by the end of 4 years, the orlistat-treated patients were −6.9% below baseline compared with −4.1% for those receiving placebo. The trial also showed a 37% reduction in the conversion of patients from impaired glucose tolerance to diabetes; essentially all of this benefit occurred in the patients with impaired glucose tolerance at enrollment into the trial. In another study of orlistat and weight loss, investigators pooled data on 675 subjects from three of the 2-year studies described previously in which glucose tolerance tests were available. During treatment, 6.6% of the patients taking orlistat converted from a normal to an impaired glucose tolerance test compared with 10.8% in the placebo-treated group. None of the orlistat-treated patients who originally had normal glucose tolerance developed diabetes compared with 1.2% in the placebo-treated group. Of those who initially had normal glucose tolerance, 7.6% in the placebo group but only 3% in the orlistat-treated group developed diabetes.

Safety

Orlistat is not absorbed to any significant degree, and its side effects are thus related to the blockade of triglyceride digestion in the intestine. Fecal fat loss and related GI symptoms are common initially, but they subside as patients learn to use the drug. The QOL in patients treated with orlistat may improve despite concerns about GI symptoms. Orlistat can cause small but significant decreases in fat-soluble vitamins. Levels usually remain within the normal range, but a few patients may need vitamin supplementation. Because it is impossible to tell which patients need vitamins, it is wise to provide a multivitamin routinely with instructions to take it before bedtime. Orlistat does not seem to affect the absorption of other drugs, except acyclovir.

Managing patients with pharmacotherapy

Pharmacotherapy should be considered only if the patient will be taking the medication in conjunction with an overall weight management program, including a reduced calorie diet and increased physical activity, and has realistic expectations of medication therapy. Successful use of anti-obesity medications still requires that patients deliberately and consciously alter their behavior for weight loss to occur. In other words, the pharmacologic action of anti-obesity medications must be *translated* into behavior change. During follow-up, body weight and vital signs should be measured and side effects and intended effects reviewed. For sympathomimetic drugs, it is important to ask the patients on the medication about their feelings of hunger and fullness. Careful notice should be given to blood pressure and heart rate, since a significant increase in either may warrant lowering the dose or discontinuing the medication entirely. For orlistat, it is important to ask the patient about GI effects and dietary intake of fat. Approximately 10–25% of patients experience a GI effect, such as oily spotting, flatus with discharge, fecal urgency, and fatty stool.

Weight-gaining medications

An iatrogenic increase in body weight occurs when medications prescribed for management of chronic diseases have the side effect of weight gain. This is most often seen with anti-diabetic, psychotropic, anti-depressant, steroid, and anti-hypertensive medications. Box 11.1 lists common offending medications that result is weight gain as a side effect. Iatrogenic weight gain is identified by taking thorough medication history. When possible, weight-gaining medications should be reduced or discontinued and replaced with non-weight-gaining medications.

Box 11.1 Medications associated with body weight gain.

Psychiatric/neurological drugs

Anti-psychotic agents: phenothiazines, olanzapine, clozapine, risperidone
    Mood stabilizers: lithium
Anti-depressants: tricyclics, MAOIs, SSRIs (paroxetine), mirtazapine
Antiepileptic drugs: gabapentin, valproate, carbamazepine

Steroid hormones

Corticosteriods
Progestational steroids

Anti-diabetes agents

Insulin, sulfonylureas, thiazolidinediones (TZDs)

Anti-hypertensive agents

Beta- and alpha-1 adrenergic receptor blockers

Antihistamines

Cyproheptadine

Pitfalls

- Prescribing anti-obesity medication without concomitant lifestyle modification will lead to less weight loss.
- Prescribing orlistat without counseling on dietary fat restrictions will lead to increased GI side effects and patient's discontinuation of medication.
- If realistic expectations are not discussed with patients, they will be disappointed with the benefits of pharmacotherapy.

Key web links

http://www.qsymia.com/ [accessed on December 29, 2012].
http://qsymia.com/pdf/prescribing-information.pdf [accessed on January 22, 2013].
http://us.eisai.com/package_inserts/BelviqPI.pdf [accessed on December 29, 2012].

Further reading

Allison, D.B., Gadde, K.M., Garvey, W.T. *et al.* (2011) Controlled-release phentermine/topiramate in severely obese adults: A randomized controlled trial (EQUIP). *Obesity,* 20, 330–342.

Astrup, A., Rossner, S., Van Gaal, L. *et al.* (2009) Effects of liraglutide in the treatment of obesity: A randomized, double-blind, placebo-controlled study. *Lancet,* 374, 1606–1616.

Fider, M.C., Sanchez, M., Raether, B. *et al.* (2011) A one-year randomized trial of lorcaserin for weight loss in obese and overweight adults: The BLOSSOM trial. *Journal of Clinical Endocrinology and Metabolism,* 96, 3067–3077.

Gadde, K.M., Allison, D.B., Ryan, D.H. *et al.* (2011) Effects of low-dose, controlled-release, phentermine plus topiramate combination on weight and associated comorbidities in overweight and obese adults (CONQUER): A randomized, placebo-controlled, phase 3 trial. *Lancet,* 377, 1341–1352.

Garvey, W.T., Ryan, D.H., Look, M. *et al.* (2012) Two-year sustained weight loss and metabolic benefits with controlled-release phentermine/topiramate in obese and overweight adults (SEQUEL): A randomized, placebo-controlled, phase 3 extension study. *American Journal of Clinical Nutrition*, 95, 297–308.

Leslie, W.S., Hankey, C.R. & Lean, M.E.J. (2007) Weight gain as an adverse effect of some commonly prescribed drugs: A systematic review. *Quarterly Journal of Medicine*, 100, 395–404.

Powell, A.G., Apovian, C.M. & Aronne, L.J. (2011) New drug targets for the treatment of obesity. *Clinical Pharmacology & Therapeutics*, 90, 40–51.

Rucker, D., Padwal, R., Li, S.K. *et al.* (2007) Long term pharmacotherapy for obesity and overweight: Updated meta-analysis. *BMJ*, 335, 1194–1199.

Smith, S.R., Weissman, N.J., Anderson, C.M. *et al.* (2010) Multicenter, placebo-controlled trial of lorcaserin for weight management. *New England Journal of Medicine*, 363, 245–256.

CHAPTER 12

Surgery

Key points

- Bariatric surgery can be considered for patients with severe obesity (BMI ≥ 40 kg/m²) or those with moderate obesity (BMI ≥ 35 kg/m²) associated with comorbid conditions.
- Weight loss surgeries fall into one of three categories: restrictive, restrictive–malabsorptive, and malabsorptive.
- Bariatric surgery is the most effective weight loss therapy for patients with clinically severe obesity.
- Post-operative care requires management of co-morbidities, dietary and lifestyle counseling, and monitoring and treatment of surgical complications.

CASE STUDIES

Case study 1

JS is a 54-year-old male with a BMI of 42 kg/m². He has progressively gained weight with each passing decade to his current and heaviest body weight. He is taking seven medications for the medical management of T2DM, hypertension, mixed hyperlipidemia, osteoarthritis, and OSA. He has previously lost between 5% and 20% of his weight through numerous professional and commercial weight loss programs; however, he is unable to maintain the weight loss long term. He is frustrated about his weight and is concerned that his QOL will continue to decline.

Comment: You inform JS that weight loss surgery is a viable option. You briefly explain how the surgical treatments work and refer him for consultation with a bariatric surgeon.

Case study 2

AD is a 42-year-old woman who underwent an uneventful laparoscopic RYGB procedure 2 years ago. She has successfully lost 44.5 kg representing 35% of her initial body weight. Her diabetes and GERD are in remission off all medications. However, she is experiencing increased fatigue and an unusual craving for ice for the

---

Practical Manual of Clinical Obesity, First Edition. Robert Kushner, Victor Lawrence and Sudhesh Kumar.
© 2013 John Wiley & Sons, Ltd. Published 2013 by John Wiley & Sons, Ltd.

past 4 months. AD takes her prescribed vitamin and mineral supplements on an intermittent basis. Laboratory testing discloses iron deficiency anemia and a low 25-hydroxy vitamin D level.

Comment: In addition to a multiple vitamin–mineral supplement, you prescribe oral iron t.i.d., vitamin B_{12}, and vitamin D with calcium.

Bariatric surgery can be considered for patients with severe obesity (BMI ≥ 40 kg/m²) or those with moderate obesity (BMI ≥ 35 kg/m²) associated with comorbid conditions. Bariatric surgery results in weight loss and improvement of multiple co-morbid conditions and is the most effective treatment for patients with severe obesity.

Weight loss procedures

Weight loss surgeries fall into one of three categories: restrictive, restrictive–malabsorptive, and malabsorptive. Although this traditional classification continues today, the mechanisms for weight loss are more complex and physiological than simply restrictive and malabsorptive factors. Restrictive surgeries limit the amount of food the stomach can hold and slow down the rate of gastric emptying. Laparoscopic adjustable gastric banding (LAGB) is the most commonly performed restrictive procedure (Figure 12.1). The two products available in the market are Lap-Band® (Allergan) and Realize®Band (EndoEthicon). The diameters of these bands are adjustable by way of their connection to a reservoir that is implanted under the skin. Injection or removal of saline into the reservoir tightens or loosens the band's internal diameter, thus changing the size of the gastric opening. Laparoscopic sleeve gastrectomy (LSG) is a relatively new option. The early reports are favorable regarding weight loss and co-morbidity outcomes, but it is unknown whether an additional procedure will be required for long-term weight loss.

The combined restrictive–malabsorptive procedure combines the elements of gastric restriction, selective malabsorption, and changes in GI hormonal responses. The most common procedure is the RYGB (Figure 12.2). It involves the formation of a 10–30-mL proximal gastric pouch by either surgically separating or stapling the stomach across the fundus. Outflow from the pouch is created by performing a narrow (10-mm) gastrojejunostomy. The distal end of jejunum is then anastomosed 50–150 cm below the gastrojejunostomy. "Roux-en-Y" refers to the Y-shaped section of the small intestine created by the surgery; the Y is created at the point where the pancreo-biliary conduit (afferent limb) and the Roux (efferent limb) are connected. "Bypass" refers to the exclusion or bypassing of the distal stomach, duodenum, and proximal jejunum.

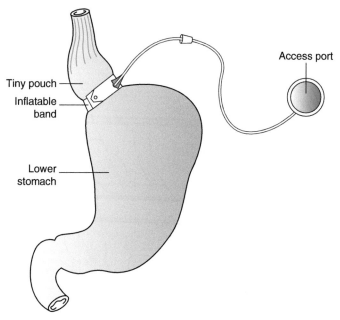

Figure 12.1 Laparoscopic adjustable gastric band (LAGB). Reproduced from Kopelman *et al. Clinical Obesity in Adults and Children*, 3rd edn, Blackwell Publishing, Oxford, 2010, with permission from Blackwell Publishing.

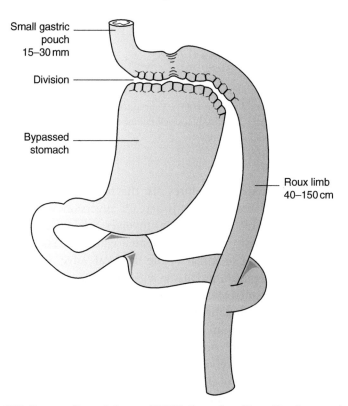

Figure 12.2 Roux-en-Y gastric bypass (RYGB). Reproduced from Kopelman *et al. Clinical Obesity in Adults and Children*, 3rd edn, Blackwell Publishing, Oxford, 2010, with permission from Blackwell Publishing.

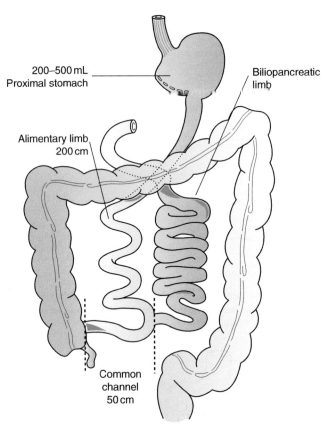

Figure 12.3 Biliopancreatic diversion (BPD). Reproduced from Kopelman *et al. Clinical Obesity in Adults and Children*, 3rd edn, Blackwell Publishing, Oxford, 2010, with permission from Blackwell Publishing.

The two malabsorptive procedures are the bilio-pancreatic diversion (BPD) (Figure 12.3) and the bilio-pancreatic diversion with duodenal switch (BPDDS) (Figure 12.4). The BPD involves a subtotal gastrectomy, leaving a much larger gastric pouch compared with the RYGB. The small bowel is divided 250 cm proximal to the ileocecal valve and connected directly to the gastric pouch, producing a gastroileostomy. The remaining proximal limb (bilio-pancreatic conduit) is then anastomosed to the side of the distal ileum 50 cm proximal to the ileocecal valve. In this procedure, the distal stomach, duodenum, and entire jejunum are bypassed, leaving only a 50-cm distal ileum common channel for nutrients to mix with pancreatic and biliary secretions. BPDDS is a variation of BPD which preserves the first portion of the duodenum. In this procedure, a vertical subtotal gastrectomy is performed and the duodenum is divided just beyond the pylorus. The distal small bowel is connected to the short stump

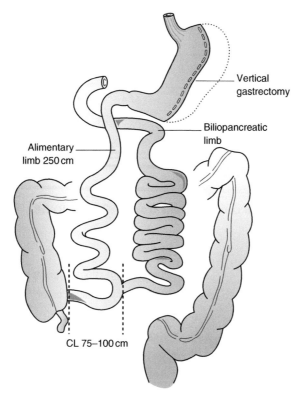

Figure 12.4 Biliopancreatic diversion with duodenal switch (BPDDS). Reproduced from Kopelman *et al. Clinical Obesity in Adults and Children*, 3rd edn, Blackwell Publishing, Oxford, 2010, with permission from Blackwell Publishing.

of the duodenum, producing a 75–100-cm ileal–duodenal "common channel" for absorption of nutrients. The other end of the duodenum is closed, and the remaining small bowel is connected onto the enteral limb at about 75–100 cm from the ileocecal valve.

Weight loss and complications

Although no recent randomized controlled trials compare weight loss after surgical and non-surgical interventions, data from meta-analyses and large databases, primarily obtained from observational studies, suggest that bariatric surgery is the most effective weight loss therapy for those with clinically severe obesity. Although total weight loss is greater with malabsorptive procedures, they are also associated with greater complication rates. Reported weight loss as percentage of excess body weight after bariatric surgery is shown in Table 12.1. Surgical mortality from bariatric surgery is

Table 12.1 Reported weight loss as percentage of excess body weight after bariatric surgery.

Study	RYGB (%)	LAGB (%)	BPD (%)	Follow-up (years)
Buchwald et al. [1], n=22,094	61.5	47.4	70.1	≤2
O'Brien et al. [2], n=1703 reports	52.5–58.2	49.8–59.3	69.0–77.0	5–10
Garb et al. [3], n=7383	61.5–71.2	42.6–55.2	–	5–7.25

Box 12.1 Potential complications from LAGB and RYGB.

Complication profiles

RYGB

- Incisional hernia
- Bowel obstruction
- Internal hernia
- Stomal stenosis
- Micronutrient deficiencies
- Marginal ulcer
- Weight regain

LAGB

- Band slippage (stomach prolapse)
- Leakage of the balloon or tubing
- Port infection
- Band infection
- Obstruction
- Band erosion into the stomach
- Esophageal dilation
- Failure to lose weight

---

generally less than 1% but varies with the procedure, patient's age, co-morbid conditions, and experience of the surgical team. An abundance of data supports the positive impact of bariatric surgery on obesity-related morbid conditions, including diabetes mellitus, hypertension, OSA, dyslipidemia, and NAFLD. Potential complications from the LAGB and RYGB are listed in Box 12.1.

Effect on co-morbid conditions

Type 2 diabetes (T2DM)

Weight loss protects obese subjects with or without impaired glucose tolerance from the development of diabetes. The RYGB procedure induces remission of T2DM in over 80% of cases and appears to have an almost immediate effect on hyperglycemia before significant weight loss has been achieved. The reason(s) for this early effect is likely to be related to the GI diversion produced by the bypass procedure. Chyme from the stomach bypasses much of the stomach, duodenum, and upper jejunum. Some believe bypass of the duodenum stimulates an incretin effect on the pancreatic β cell, stimulating insulin secretion (the foregut hypothesis), and others suggest that the premature delivery of food into the distal small bowel also has an incretin effect, possibly due to glucagon-like peptide-1 secretion from the mucosal L-cells (hindgut hypothesis). The exact clinical relevance and the durability of this early glycemic control are unknown.

Importantly, improvement in diabetes following weight loss is related to the dual effects of improvement in insulin sensitivity and pancreatic β cell function. As β cell function deteriorates progressively over time in those with T2DM, early weight loss intervention should therefore be a central part of initial therapy in severely obese subjects who develop T2DM. For obese patients with T2DM, weight loss provides benefit unequaled by any other therapy and may prove to be the only therapy that substantially changes the natural history of the disease.

Dyslipidemia of obesity

Increased fasting triglyceride and decreased HDL-cholesterol concentrations characterize the dyslipidemia of obesity and insulin resistance. Weight loss surgery produces substantial decreases in fasting triglyceride levels, an elevation of HDL-cholesterol levels to normal, and an improved total cholesterol to HDL cholesterol ratio. Although elevation of total cholesterol is not a feature of obesity, hypercholesterolemia can be controlled by malabsorptive procedures such as BPD and RYGB.

Hypertension

Improvements in hypertension are frequently seen following all types of bariatric surgery. Non-diuretic anti-hypertensive medications are not typically discontinued in the immediate post-operative period; therefore, it is unclear how quickly this benefit occurs. A number of studies have demonstrated positive effects on blood pressure 1–2 years after bariatric surgery. Buchwald and colleagues found that 62% of surgical patients had resolution of hypertension, a finding that appeared to be independent of surgical procedure. There is some evidence to suggest, however, that this benefit may not persist long term. A case series of over 1000 gastric bypass patients demonstrated resolution of high blood pressure (defined as blood pressure less than 135/85 in the absence of anti-hypertensive medications) in 69% of patients 1–2 years after surgery. By 10–12 years post-op, however, this number had dropped to 51%. In the Swedish Obese Subjects (SOS) study, the incidence of hypertension (blood pressure ≥ 140/90) did not differ between surgery and control groups at 2 and 10 years, but recovery from hypertension was more frequent in the surgery group at both points in time.

Obstructive sleep apnea (OSA)

Obstructive sleep apnea (OSA) is common in obese individuals. Bariatric surgery has been shown to have a positive effect on this condition as well. A recent systematic literature review noted improvement in OSA in a number of studies that evaluated patients after both RYGB and LAGB. Buchwald and colleagues' meta-analysis showed striking results, with over 85% of patients having complete resolution of the disorder. These authors also reported data from a sub-analysis of four studies (92 subjects) that showed a mean decrease of 33.9 apneas or hypopneas per hour after bariatric surgery.

Changes in QOL after bariatric surgery

Improvement in QOL is one of the most gratifying outcomes of bariatric surgery. A number of studies clearly demonstrate major QOL improvements following LAGB and other procedures. In a study of 459 severely obese subjects reported by O'Brien and Dixon who measured QOL after LAGB with the Medical Outcomes Trust Short Form-36 (SF-36), severely obese subjects had lower scores compared with community normal values for all eight aspects of QOL measured, especially the physical health scores. LAGB provided a dramatic and sustained improvement in all measures of SF-36. Improvement was greater in those with more pre-operative disability, and the extent of weight loss was not a good predictor of improved QOL. Mean scores returned to those of community normal values by 1 year after surgery and remained in the normal range throughout the 4 years of the study.

Patient selection and pre-operative management

Patients who meet the criteria listed in Box 12.2 should be considered for bariatric surgery. Patients should be evaluated by a multidisciplinary team of health professionals that include (at a minimum) a physician, registered dietitian, and clinical psychologist. Pre-operative management should include risk reduction, education, and behavior change. In the USA, referral to a bariatric center of excellence as designated by the American College of Surgeons Bariatric Surgery Center Network (ACS BSCN) accreditation program (ascbscn.org/Public/index.jsp) should be considered to reduce operative morbidity and mortality.

Post-operative management

Post-operative care requires management of co-morbidities, dietary and lifestyle counseling, and monitoring and treatment of surgical complications. Anti-diabetic and anti-hypertensive medications are typically

---

Box 12.2 Criteria to be met for consideration for bariatric surgery.

Surgical treatment

Who should be considered?

• BMI of ≥40 kg/m² or ≥35 kg/m² with co-morbidity

• Unable to achieve and maintain healthier body weight with non-surgical approaches

• A well-informed and motivated patient

• Has a strong social support system

• Acceptable operative risks

• No significant mental health problems that would preclude post-operative compliance or may worsen after surgery

---

Table 12.2 Routine nutrient supplementation after bariatric surgery.

Supplement	Dose
MVI	1–2 daily
Ca-citrate with added vitamin D	1200–2000 mg/day + 2000 unit/day
Folic acid	400 µg/day in MVI
Elemental iron[b]	40–65 mg/day
Vitamin B₁₂	≥350 µg/day
	or 1000 µg/month IM
	or 3000 µg q 6 month IM
	or 500 µg q week intranasal

Source: Mechanick *et al*. [4].
MVI, multivitamin; Ca, calcium; IM, intramuscular.
[a] Patients with pre- or post-operative biochemical deficiency states are treated beyond these recommendations.
[b] In women who menstruate, vitamin C.

reduced depending on the patient's response to surgery. Other medications should be adjusted as needed. Patients are guided through advancing meal progressions over the first 6 weeks with the assistance of a registered dietitian. For patients who undergo LAGB, there are no intestinal absorptive abnormalities other than mechanical reductions in gastric size and outflow. Therefore, selective deficiencies occur uncommonly unless eating habits become unbalanced. In contrast, the restrictive–malabsorptive procedures increase risk for micronutrient deficiencies of vitamin B_{12}, iron, folate, calcium, and vitamin D. Patients with restrictive–malabsorptive procedures require lifelong supplementation with these micronutrients. Recommended supplements are shown in Table 12.2. The most common surgical complications include stomal stenosis and marginal ulcers (occurring in 5–15% of patients) that present as prolonged nausea and vomiting after eating or inability to advance the diet to solid foods. These complications are typically treated by endoscopic balloon dilatation and acid suppression therapy, respectively.

Pitfalls

- Considering bariatric surgery only as the treatment of last resort may extend progression of obesity-related co-morbidities.
- Not monitoring the predictable malabsorption of vitamins and minerals that may occur following malabsorptive surgery will lead to subclinical and clinical deficiencies.
- Infrequent or inadequate post-operative follow-up may lead to less successful weight loss outcomes.

Key web links

http://www.uptodate.com/contents/weight-loss-surgery-beyond-the-basics?view=print [accessed on December 29, 2012].
http://www.mayoclinic.com/health/gastric-bypass/MY00825/METHOD=print [accessed on December 29, 2012].
http://www.lapband.com/en/home [accessed on December 29, 2012].
http://www.realize.com/ [accessed on December 29, 2012].

References

1 Buchwald, H., Avidor, Y., Braunwald, E. *et al.* (2004) Bariatric surgery. A systematic review and meta-analysis. *Journal of American Medical Association*, 292, 1724–1737.
2 O'Brien, P.E., McPhail, T., Chaston, T.B. & Dixon, J.B. (2006) Systematic review of medium-term weight loss after bariatric operations. *Obesity Surgery*, 6, 1032–1040.
3 Garb, J., Welch, G., Zagarins, S., Kuhn, J. & Romanelli, J. (2009) Bariatric surgery for the treatment of morbid obesity: A meta-analysis of weight loss outcomes for laparoscopic adjustable gastric banding and laparoscopic gastric bypass. *Obesity Surgery*, 19, 1447–1455.
4 Mechanick, J.I., Kushner, R.F., Sugerman, H.J. & For the Writing Group. (2009) AACE/TOS/ASMBS Guidelines. American Association of Clinical Endocrinologists, Obesity Society, and American Society for Metabolic & Bariatric Surgery medical guidelines for clinical practice for the perioperative nutritional, metabolic, and nonsurgical support of the bariatric surgery patient. *Obesity* 17 (Suppl. 1), S1–S70.

Further reading

Aills, L., Blankenship, J., Buffington, C., Furtado, M. & Parrott, J. (2008) ASMBS Allied Health nutritional guidelines for the surgical weight loss patient. *Surgery for Obesity and Related Diseases*, 4, S73–S108.

Carlsson, L.M.S., Peltonen, M., Ahlin, S. *et al.* (2012) Bariatric surgery and prevention of type 2 diabetes in Swedish Obese Subjects. *New England Journal of Medicine*, 367, 695–704.

Fried, M., Hainer, V., Basdevant, A. *et al.* (2007) Inter-disciplinary European guidelines on surgery of severe obesity. *International Journal of Obesity*, 31, 569–577.

Heber, D., Greenway, F.L., Kaplan, L.M., Livingston, E., Salvador, J. & Still, C. (2010) Endocrine and nutritional management of the post-bariatric surgery patient: An endocrine society clinical practice guideline. *Journal of Clinical Endocrinology and Metabolism*, 95, 4823–4843.

Ochner, C.N., Gibson, C., Shanik, M., Goel, V. & Geliebter, A. (2011) Changes in neuro-hormonal gut peptides following bariatric surgery. *International Journal of Obesity*, 35, 153–166.

Sauerland, S., Angrisani, L., Belachew, M. *et al.* (2005) Evidence-based guidelines of the European Association for Endoscopic Surgery (EAES). Obesity surgery. *Surgical Endoscopy*, 19, 200–221.

Clinical Management of Obesity-Related Co-morbidities

Sudhesh Kumar and Milan K. Piya,
Section Editors

CHAPTER 13

Diabetes and Metabolic Diseases

Key points

- A small amount of weight loss (5–7%) is associated with clinical improvements in glycemic and metabolic control in patients with obesity and T2DM.

- When selecting medication management for patients with T2DM and obesity, the beneficial effects on body weight should be strongly considered along with glycemic control.

- In the obese patient with T2DM, look for associated cardio-metabolic risk factors, such as hypertension, dyslipidemia, NAFLD, and OSA.

- In the obese patient with pre-diabetes or T2DM, consider active weight loss management at every stage of the disease. Many associated co-morbidities will also improve with weight loss.

- The poorly controlled severely obese patient with T2DM may benefit from bariatric surgery to reduce risk factors.

CASE STUDIES

Case study 1

LK is a 52-year-old bank executive who has been putting on weight steadily over the last 6 years. She attributes the weight gain to spending more time at work and lack of sleep. Her weight has now reached 210 lb with a BMI of 36 kg/m². Her fasting blood glucose was 155 mg/dL and hemoglobin A1c (HbA1c) was 7.2%. Her triglyceride and HDL-cholesterol levels were 250 and 38 mg/dL, respectively.

Comment: She was placed on metformin 850 mg b.i.d. and was prescribed a 1400-kcal diet that included carbohydrates from fruits, vegetables, whole grains, and legumes. She increased her physical activity to 30 min of brisk walking 5 days/week. After 3 months of lifestyle modification, she successfully lost 10 lb. Repeat fasting blood glucose and HbA1c were 120 mg/dL and 6.2%, respectively.

Case study 2

PH, a 30-year-old male taxi driver, had T2DM for 3 years. He had been putting on weight and admitted to eating a lot of fast food and not doing any exercise. His BMI

Practical Manual of Clinical Obesity, First Edition. Robert Kushner, Victor Lawrence and Sudhesh Kumar.

> was 43 kg/m² and his diabetes control was poor with an HbA1c of 9.2% despite taking four types of medication including gliclazide, metformin, pioglitazone, and sitagliptin. He was reluctant to start insulin for fear of hypoglycemia and the effect on his driving license, and he opted for bariatric surgery.
>
> **Comment:** After undergoing an RYGB procedure, he was able to discontinue all of his anti-diabetic medication within 1 week and achieved an HbA1c of 6.5% by 6 months. He remains in diabetes remission after 1 year along with a 30% reduction in total body weight.

Principles guiding management

Obesity, fat distribution, and diabetes

Estimates of the prevalence of obesity in patients with T2DM vary between 60% and 90% depending on age and ethnicity. The combination of the two conditions has been referred to as "diabesity." The incidence of T2DM is related to increased BMI, weight gain, and body fat distribution. Waist circumference, particularly when combined with other measures of insulin resistance, such as elevated serum triglyceride concentration (greater than 150 mg/dL), a low HDL-cholesterol concentration (less than 40 mg/dL), or a high triglyceride–HDL cholesterol ratio (greater than 3), is a good predictor of the risk of the metabolic syndrome in the obese individual. The "cutoffs" for abnormal waist circumference are shown in Table 13.1.

Obesity, ethnicity, and diabetes

The recent epidemic of T2DM affects virtually all populations, with particularly high rates seen in South Asian diaspora and also Black and Hispanic populations in western Europe and North America. There have been large increases in the number of people developing diabetes in low- and middle-income countries of Asia and Africa as well. A particularly troubling development is the appearance of T2DM in the pediatric population, reflecting the increasing prevalence of obesity in this group. There are now ethnicity-specific criteria for diagnosis and management of obesity in ethnic minorities (Table 13.1).

Obesity and the "metabolic syndrome"

The metabolic syndrome, also known as syndrome X, is a complex set of traits that cluster together and enhance the risk of CVD. It includes a variety of factors, including central obesity, elevated blood pressure, insulin resistance, dyslipidemia, and elevated blood glucose. In an effort to provide a unified definition of this syndrome, a joint statement from IDF, National Heart Lung and Blood institute (NHLBI), American Heart Association (AHA), World Heart Federation, International Atherosclerosis Society, and

Table 13.1 Ethnicity-specific values for waist circumference.

Country/ethnic group	Waist circumference
Europids	
In the USA, the ATP III values (102 cm male; 88 cm female) are likely to continue to be used for clinical purposes	
Male	≥94 cm
Female	≥80 cm
South Asians	
Based on a Chinese, Malay, and Asian-Indian population	
Male	≥90 cm
Female	≥80 cm
Chinese	
Male	≥90 cm
Female	≥80 cm
Japanese	
Male	≥90 cm
Female	≥80 cm
Ethnic South and Central Americans	
Use South Asian recommendations until more specific data are available	
Sub-Saharan Africans	
Use European data until more specific data are available	
Eastern Mediterranean and Middle East (Arab) populations	
Use European data until more specific data are available	

Central obesity is most easily measured by waist circumference using the guidelines in Table 13.1, which are gender and ethnic group (not country of residence) specific. The consensus group acknowledges that these are pragmatic cut points taken from various different data sources and that better data will be needed to link these to risk.

International Association for the Study of Obesity has provided defining features (Table 13.2). The syndrome is associated with abdominal obesity, measured in this definition by waist circumference. Like BMI itself, abdominal fat and its risks vary in different ethnic populations and need ethnic sensitivity in their interpretation. For example, measurements of insulin resistance suggest that individuals of Asian descent (Chinese, Japanese, and South Indians) may have more abdominal fat for a given BMI and body fat than Caucasians. Patients with diabetes are at a high risk of future CVD, but these criteria help to identify individuals without diabetes who are at a high risk of developing cardiovascular complications. However, more accurate predictions of risk can be made using various cardiovascular

Table 13.2 IDF criteria for diagnosis of metabolic syndrome.

Central obesity (defined as waist circumference[a] ≥ 94 cm for Europid men and ≥ 80 cm for Europid women, with ethnicity-specific values for other groups) plus any two of the following four factors:

- Raised triglyceride level: ≥150 mg/dL (1.7 mmol/L), or specific treatment for this lipid abnormality
- Reduced HDL cholesterol: less than 40 mg/dL (1.03 mmol/L*) in males and less than 50 mg/dL (1.29 mmol/L*) in females, or specific treatment for this lipid abnormality
- Raised blood pressure: systolic BP ≥ 130 or diastolic BP ≥ 85 mmHg, or treatment of previously diagnosed hypertension
- Raised fasting plasma glucose (FPG) ≥ 100 mg/dL (5.6 mmol/L), or previously diagnosed T2DM. If above 5.6 mmol/L or 100 mg/dL, oral glucose tolerance test (OGTT) is strongly recommended but is not necessary to define presence of the syndrome

---

[a] If BMI is greater than 30 kg/m², central obesity can be assumed and waist circumference does not need to be measured.

risk scores, such as the Framingham risk score or the United Kingdom Prospective Diabetes Study (UKPDS) risk engine.

Obesity management and control of cardiovascular risk factors

A key point to emphasize in the care of the overweight patient with T2DM is that weight loss should be considered the primary treatment strategy along with medication management to control hypertension, dyslipidemia, and hyperglycemia to achieve therapeutic targets. This paradigm shift from a "glucose-centered" to an "obesity-centered" view of management is supported by the beneficial effects of weight loss on reductions in blood glucose, blood pressure, mixed hyperlipidemia, and fatty liver disease.

Lifestyle modification for the obese pre-diabetic and diabetic patient

Lifestyle modification is the cornerstone of treatment for pre-diabetes and T2DM. It encompasses prescription of a hypocaloric diet, increased physical activity and exercise, and changes in self-care behavior. Reductions in HbA1c of 1–2% can be expected depending upon the patient's initial glycemic control and habitual diet. The optimal macronutrient distribution of weight loss diets has not been established. For weight loss, either low-carbohydrate or low-fat calorie-restricted diets may be effective. Whereas low-carbohydrate diets are associated with improvements in triglyceride and HDL-cholesterol concentrations compared to low-fat diets, LDL cholesterol may be adversely affected by low-carbohydrate diets.

The US National Institutes of Health (NIH) Diabetes Prevention Program (DPP) and the Action for Health in Diabetes (Look AHEAD) are two landmark studies that have addressed the efficacy of lifestyle modification in reducing the risk of developing diabetes among high-risk individuals and among patients with existing T2DM, respectively.

The hypothesis of the DPP was that a 7% reduction in initial weight, combined with increased physical activity, would reduce the risk of developing T2DM in at-risk individuals. Between 1996 and 1999, 3234 patients, aged 50.6 ± 10.7 years with a BMI of 34.0 ± 6.7 and impaired glucose tolerance, were randomly assigned to placebo, metformin 850 mg b.i.d., or lifestyle intervention. Components of the individualized lifestyle intervention included a reduction in dietary fat and energy intake by 500–1000 kcal/day, exercise at least 150 min/week, self-recording, and setting realistic goals for weight loss and behavior change. After 3.3 years of follow-up, the risk of new-onset diabetes was reduced by 58% and 31% by the lifestyle and metformin groups, respectively, compared to placebo. Post hoc analysis suggested that, for every kilogram of weight loss, there was a 16% reduction in the risk of diabetes, adjusted for change in diet and activity. Prevention or delay of diabetes with lifestyle intervention or metformin persisted up to 10 years.

A demonstrated beneficial effect of lifestyle modification on the development of diabetes was the impetus for the design of the Look AHEAD trial. The hypothesis of this trial was that a loss of 7% or more of initial body weight with increased physical activity will reduce the risk of cardiovascular morbidity and mortality in overweight and obese persons with T2DM followed over 13.5 years. In this multicenter, controlled trial, launched in 2001, 5145 overweight subjects with T2DM were randomized into two arms: usual care (diabetes support and education (DSE)) and usual care plus intensive lifestyle intervention (ILI). In contrast to the DPP study, subjects in Look AHEAD were slightly older (58.7 ± 6.8 years) and heavier (BMI 36.0 ± 6.0). Differences in intervention included seeing participants in groups and individually, the exercise goal was raised to 175 min/week, subjects counted calories instead of fat grams, and meal replacement products were prescribed to replace two meals and one snack daily for the first 4 months and reduced use thereafter. For the first year, ILI subjects attended—two to three group sessions and one individual session per month. The DSE subjects attended three meetings per year to promote retention.

At 1 year, subjects in the ILI group lost 8.6 ± 6.9% of initial weight compared to a significantly smaller 0.7 ± 4.8% for individuals in DSE. The mean HbA1c level dropped from 7.3% to 6.6% in ILI versus from 7.3% to 7.2% in DSE. Over 19% of the variability in weight loss in the ILI group was predicted by three variables: minutes of physical activity, attendance at sessions, and inclusion of meal replacements. After 4 years of follow-up, mean percent weight loss in the ILI and DSE groups remained significantly different (−6.15% vs −0.88%), along with continued improvements in the HbA1c level (−0.36% vs −0.09%) and other cardiovascular risk factors. Whether these differences in weight loss and risk factors translate into reduction in CVD events after 13.5 years of follow-up is yet to be determined. Nonetheless, data thus far support the beneficial effect of ILI in patients at risk for diabetes or who have existing diabetes.

Management algorithm

Maintaining glycemic control during weight management

Drug therapy for T2DM and associated cardiovascular risk factors is proven to reduce long-term complications, such as CVD and microvascular complications. Therefore, it is important to aim for good control of diabetes and associated risk factors by optimally using available drugs.

Early in the course of diabetes, when metformin alone or insulin-sparing drugs can be used, it is appropriate to aim for tight glycemic control reflected in an HbA1c of 6.5% or lower. Once three or more drugs are required or if insulin is required, the target HbA1c recommended is 7.5%. Early tight control of glycemia is also thought to produce a legacy effect with long-term benefits accruing long after the initial period of tight control, as shown in the long-term follow-up data of the UKPDS.

Choice of drugs

Insulin-sparing drugs tend to avoid hyperinsulinemia and include agents that are weight neutral or result in weight loss. Unless not tolerated due to GI side effects or contra-indicated due to impaired renal function (increased risk of lactic acidosis), metformin is the first-line therapy in T2DM since metformin is weight neutral and improves long-term outcomes in diabetes, as shown in the UKPDS trial. DPP-4 inhibitors (sitagliptin, vildagliptin, saxagliptin and linagliptin) are also weight neutral and can be used in addition to metformin. Other agents such as sulfonylureas, meglitinides, and TZDs as well as insulin therapy are options that may promote weight gain. TZDs should be avoided if there is risk of heart failure or fluid overload. Initiation and intensification of insulin therapy should be combined with metformin to mitigate weight gain. Table 13.2 shows average weight gain with various medications for patients with T2DM. The effect on the individual patient will depend on the initial HbA1c, body weight, as well as degree of patient compliance with diet and exercise advice.

Incretin mimetics (e.g., exenatide, liraglutide and lixisenatide) are injectable GLP-1 analogs that act on GLP-1 receptors. They improve beta-cell function and glycemic control while at the same time promoting weight loss. A recent

24-month study of liraglutide (randomized, double-blind, placebo-controlled 20-week study with a 2-year extension) in obese subjects demonstrated that completers who received 2.4/3.0 mg by daily injection maintained a 2-year weight loss of 7.8 kg from screening that was associated with improvements in cardiovascular risk factors.

A review of the full list of prescribed medications is important with the aim to reduce use or substitute use of any drug that may aggravate weight gain or impede weight loss. The potential for benefit of each medication must be weighed against the tendency to produce weight gain.

Bariatric surgery for patients with severe obesity and T2DM

Bariatric surgery has been shown to improve glycemic control in T2DM, leading to resolution of the disease in a large proportion of patients. In a recent meta-analysis by Buchwald *et al.* that included a database of 621 studies, T2DM was resolved in 75% of patients ≥2 years after undergoing bariatric surgery. In general, recovery of diabetes is greatest with the malabsorptive procedure (BPD) followed by the restrictive–malabsorptive procedure (RYGB) than with the restrictive procedures (laparoscopic gastric banding and gastric sleeve). Although the mechanisms of bariatric surgery on T2DM remain unclear, the factors that support resolution include reduced carbohydrate intake, prolonged weight loss, increased insulin sensitivity, earlier release of GLP-1 (an incretin hormone) from the ileal L-cells, and exclusion of nutrients from the proximal intestine. Predictors of recurrence of diabetes are the use of insulin pre-operatively and the duration of disease. Since the long-term outcome for diabetes control remains uncertain, all patients with T2DM who undergo bariatric surgery require lifelong surveillance of blood glucose and HbA1c.

Managing the obese patient without diabetes presenting with a metabolic abnormality

All patients with a BMI ≥ 25 kg/m² associated with other risk factors, for example, family history of diabetes, high-risk race/ethnicity, history of CVD, and women who delivered a large baby or who were diagnosed with GDM should be tested for diabetes.

Similarly, patients presenting with other risk factors for CVD (hypertension and dyslipidemia) or elevated hepatic transaminase levels (suggestive of fatty liver disease) should have a fasting blood glucose and HbA1c obtained.

Obese patient with diabetes presenting with sub-optimally controlled diabetes

Tight glycemic control is desirable at early stages of T2DM when lifestyle management can avoid progression to requiring drugs that may cause side effects such as hypoglycemia and weight gain. Insulin-sparing anti-diabetic drugs such as metformin should be used in preference, as they do not promote weight gain. There is a real opportunity at this stage for patients to lose weight through major lifestyle changes. Orlistat is the only licensed drug available at this time and can be considered. GLP-1 antagonists such as exenatide and liraglutide may be used as per license as diabetes progresses and may help with control of diabetes together with weight loss. Nausea, vomiting, and diarrhea are potential side effects with this class of drugs. When patients with T2DM present with moderate to severe obesity (BMI > 35 kg/m²) and failure to respond to medical management, bariatric surgery can be considered a therapeutic option. Bariatric surgery is discussed in detail in Chapter 12.

Pitfalls

1. Good glycemic control is important when managing obesity in patients with diabetes. Despite the fact that it may cause weight gain, insulin may be the best option for obtaining good glycemic control until patients lose weight through other interventions.
2. It is difficult to motivate people to make changes in lifestyle to lose weight. Simply providing information to patients does not always result in action.
3. Avoid orlistat when it is clear that the patient is unlikely to make significant changes in diet, particularly cutting down fat intake. The combination of orlistat and metformin is associated with more GI side effects.
4. Treatment with GLP-1 antagonists in patients taking anti-hypoglycemic drugs does not always result in weight loss. Response in terms of diabetes control and weight loss will vary. Cut doses of drugs that may cause hypoglycemia in anticipation but follow up the patient to monitor response.
5. When weight loss occurs, check that it is intentional weight loss, as many malignancies are more common in obese patients with diabetes.

Key web links

NICE Guidelines for the Management of Type 2 Diabetes. www.nice.org.uk/cg66 [accessed on December 29, 2012].

Nice Guidelines for Obesity. http://guidance.nice.org.uk/CG43 [accessed on December 29, 2012].

American Diabetes Association website. http://www.diabetes.org [accessed on December 29, 2012].

Diabetes UK website. http://www.diabetes.org.uk [accessed on December 29, 2012].

Scottish Intercollegiate Guidelines Network (SIGN) Guidelines for Obesity. http://www.sign.ac.uk/guidelines/fulltext/115/index.html [accessed on December 29, 2012].

Evidence-Based Nutrition Principles and Recommendations for the Treatment and Prevention of Diabetes and Related Complications. http://care.diabetesjournals.org/content/25/1/148.full [accessed on December 29, 2012].

http://www.idf.org/metabolic-syndrome [accessed on December 29, 2012].

References

Barnett, A.H. & Kumar, S. (ed) (2009) *Obesity and Diabetes*, 2nd edn. Wiley-Blackwell, Oxford.

Look AHEAD Research Group, Pi-Sunyer, X., Blackburn, G. *et al.* (2007) Reduction in weight and cardiovascular disease risk factors in individuals with type 2 diabetes: One-year results of the look AHEAD trial. *Diabetes Care*, 30, 1374–1383.

Further reading

Andrews R.C., Cooper, A.R., Montgomery, A.A. *et al.* (2011) Diet or diet plus physical activity versus usual care in patients with newly diagnosed type 2 diabetes: The Early ACTID randomised controlled trial. *Lancet*, 378, 129–139.

Després, J.P., Moorjani, S., Lupien, P.J., Tremblay, A., Nadeau, A. & Bouchard, C. (1992) Genetic aspects of susceptibility to obesity and related dyslipidemias. *Molecular and Cellular Biochemistry*, 113, 151–169.

Look AHEAD Research Group & Wing, R.R. (2010) Long-term effects of a lifestyle intervention on weight and cardiovascular risk factors in individuals with type 2 diabetes mellitus: Four-year results of the Look AHEAD trial. *Archives of Internal Medicine*, 170, 1566–1575.

Mokdad, A.H., Ford, E.S., Bowman, B.A. *et al.* (2003) Marks, prevalence of obesity, diabetes, and obesity-related health risk factors, 2001. *Journal of American Medical Association*, 289, 76–79.

Pories, W.J., Swanson, M.S., MacDonald, K.G. *et al.* (1995) Who would have thought it? An operation proves to be the most effective therapy for adult-onset diabetes mellitus. *Annals of Surgery*, 222, 339–352.

Sjöström, L., Narbro, K., Sjöström, C.D. *et al.* (2007) Effects of bariatric surgery on mortality in Swedish obese subjects. *New England Journal of Medicine*, 357:741–752.

Steven, M. & Haffner, L. (2006) Relationship of metabolic risk factors and development of cardiovascular disease and diabetes. *Obesity*, 14, 121S–127S.

Van Gaal, F., Mertens, I.L. & De Block, C.E. (2006) Mechanisms linking obesity with cardiovascular disease. *Nature*, 444, 875–880.

CHAPTER 14

Obesity and Reproductive Health

Key points

- Obesity is associated with PCOS and affects fertility in women.
- Obese women have poorer pregnancy outcomes. They are at higher risk of metabolic complications like diabetes both during and after pregnancy.
- All of the aforementioned poorer health outcomes due to obesity can be improved by modest weight loss. In the case of improving fertility in women with PCOS, as little as 5% weight loss may be all it takes to improve menstrual cycles and ovulatory cycles.
- Obesity is a risk factor for venous thromboembolism during treatment with estrogen-containing medication and during pregnancy.

CASE STUDIES

Case study 1

AW, a 34-year-old nurse with a BMI of 33 kg/m², was concerned that she was having irregular periods and despite not using contraception had failed to conceive over the last 3 years. She had also noticed excess body hair that was distressing. Laboratory investigations showed an increased level of LH and female testosterone levels, which confirmed the diagnosis of PCOS.

Comment: She was placed on a modest calorie-restricted diet with regular daily exercise and over the next 4 months managed to lose just over 5% of her body weight. She was planning for assisted reproduction, but to her delight, she achieved pregnancy without medical intervention. During pregnancy she was diagnosed to have gestational diabetes and required intensive insulin therapy. She delivered a 9.5- pound baby at 39 weeks. Her post-natal glucose tolerance test revealed impaired glucose tolerance.

Case study 2

SD, a 34-year-old secretary, was devastated when she had a miscarriage at 8 weeks following a pregnancy that she had been trying for several years. She had a BMI of 44

Practical Manual of Clinical Obesity, First Edition. Robert Kushner, Victor Lawrence and Sudhesh Kumar.
© 2013 John Wiley & Sons, Ltd. Published 2013 by John Wiley & Sons, Ltd.

kg/m² and attended a medical clinic to lose weight when she realized that obesity increased the risk of pregnancy loss.

Comment: She managed to lose 7 lb with lifestyle changes and went on to have a gastric band and lost over 30 lb. The following year she achieved pregnancy and delivered a healthy boy.

Obesity and reproductive health

Obesity affects myriad aspects of reproductive health. In girls, it leads to earlier menarche (or in some cases delayed menarche) and increases the risk of developing PCOS. Pregnancy in the obese is associated with the great risk of miscarriages and also a higher risk of maternal death together with a higher risk of poorer outcomes for the fetus. In men, obesity may affect fertility, and there is evidence of both hypogonadism and ED.

Obesity and menstrual disorders

Obesity affects age of onset of menarche, and the increasing prevalence of obesity in girls means that there is earlier age of onset of menarche, but reproductive performance declines earlier in obese women. Menstrual disturbances are the most common manifestation of hypothalamic–pituitary–gonadal axis dysfunction in obese women, extending from dysmenorrhea and dysfunctional uterine bleeding to amenorrhea. These abnormalities are attributed to altered androgen, estrogen, and progesterone levels, together with changes in leptin signaling in the brain. What is significant here is that even modest weight loss (as little as 5%) may restore regular menstrual cycles and ovulation.

Polycystic ovarian syndrome (PCOS)

This is a common endocrine disorder associated with obesity and is affecting an ever-increasing number of women. Obesity-associated hyperinsulinemia drives both ovarian androgen overproduction and abnormal follicular development, leading to dysfunctional uterine bleeding and anovulatory cycles. Obesity-associated fall in circulating SHBG aggravates hyperandrogenism as it leads to higher free androgen activity. Symptoms of PCOS include hirsutism, acne, and alopecia, which is often a presenting complaint. Alternatively, patients may present with infertility or dysfunctional uterine bleeding. The diagnosis of PCOS has been the subject of considerable debate, but current accepted practice is based upon the presence of two out of three criteria following a consensus meeting (known as the Rotterdam criteria). These include (1) polycystic ovaries, (2) oligo- or anovulation, and (3) clinical and/or biochemical signs of hyperandrogenism. When fertility is

Table 14.1 Complications associated with obesity in pregnancy

---

Mother

Early pregnancy
  Spontaneous abortion (miscarriage)
  Recurrent miscarriages
  Congenital anomalies
    Neural tube defects
    Spina bifida
    Congenital heart disease
  Omphalocele

Late pregnancy
  Hypertensive disorders of pregnancy
  Pre-eclampsia
  GDM
  Pre-term birth
  Intra-uterine fetal demise (stillbirth)

Peripartum
  Cesarean delivery
  Operative morbidity

Baby
  Fetal macrosomia
  Shoulder dystocia
  Childhood obesity

---

desired, obesity may complicate treatment especially in the older patients. Venous thromboembolism is a risk with estrogen (such as the combined contraceptive pill) and ovulation induction drugs like clomiphene citrate, and such therapy needs to be managed by a specialist.

Obesity and pregnancy

Increasing prevalence of obesity in the general population is also reflected in increasing numbers of pregnant women with class III obesity (BMI > 40 kg/m^2). Obesity in pregnancy is associated with a greater risk of complications for mother and baby, and therefore weight loss in such patients should be aimed for before any treatment for sub-fertility is offered (Table 14.1). Ultrasound examinations can be more difficult technically in these patients, and there could be difficulties during delivery, whether vaginal or caesarian. These patients are also at higher risk of pregnancy-induced hypertension and diabetes and, therefore, need careful monitoring. Macrosomia is a problem in many and could reflect hyperinsulinemia related to mild degrees of dysglycemia not currently treated in apparently non-diabetic obese patients. Venous thromboembolism is also more common in obese women during pregnancy.

Managing PCOS

Patients with PCOS desire improvements in many clinical parameters including fertility and regular menstrual cycles with reduction in dysfunctional uterine bleeding, reduction in hirsutism, and also improvement in co-morbid metabolic conditions. Weight loss, even modest amounts such as 5% body weight, can restore regular menstrual cycles and restore ovulation. However, as with weight loss in patients with diabetes, individuals with PCOS typically find it harder to lose weight. It is important for the treating physician to show empathy toward the patient when dealing with these sensitive issues. There is a paucity of available evidence for use of particular diets, but use of low-glycemic-index carbohydrates in preference to refined carbohydrates and modest caloric restriction with regular exercise should be recommended in these patients. Metformin is useful for improving menstrual cycles and should also be offered when the patient also has diabetes or has a dysglycemic syndrome (impaired fasting glucose or impaired glucose tolerance). For improvement of fertility, clomiphene citrate alone or in combination with metformin has been shown to be more effective than metformin alone, with the live-birth rate of combination therapy in women with infertility in PCOS as high as 26%.

Obesity and assisted reproduction therapy (ART)

Obesity impairs the outcome of ART

Other than ovulatory dysfunction, obese women are characterized by blunted responsiveness to pharmacologic treatments to induce ovulation, recurrent miscarriages, and more frequent early pregnancy loss. Crucially, reduction in weight appears to improve these outcomes. Obesity with a BMI greater than 35 kg/m^2 has been shown to reduce the probability of achieving successful live birth by 30–50%. Therefore, it is imperative that weight loss is encouraged before attempting ART. This requires considerable tact on the part of the physician as these individuals have often tried to lose weight before unsuccessfully.

Managing the pregnant obese woman

Management of obesity with clinically meaningful weight loss should be instituted before pregnancy to improve pregnancy outcomes. However, it is not uncommon to find women who have become pregnant following moderate weight loss. Management of the pregnant obese woman should

Table 14.2 IOM recommendations on weight gain during pregnancy.

Pre-pregnancy BMI	BMI+ (kg/m²) (WHO)	Total weight gain range (lb)	Rates of weight gain second and third trimester (mean range in lb/week)
Underweight	<18.5	28–40	1 (1–1.3)
Normal weight	18.5–24.9	25–35	1 (0.8–1)
Overweight	25.0–29.9	15–25	0.6 (0.5–0.7)
Obese (includes all classes)	≥30.0	11–20	0.5 (0.4–0.6)

be done with early involvement of the obstetric team. A healthy diet and regular physical exercise are beneficial to the growing fetus, and this is a factor that could motivate the mother to adopt a healthy lifestyle. In obese women, modification of unhealthy lifestyle and mitigation of associated risk factors should be implemented before, or early in, a pregnancy. Increased physical activity in women who are sedentary may result in a better pregnancy outcome for both mother and child (Table 14.2). Exercise in pregnancy may reduce pregnancy complications such as gestational diabetes and is not associated with premature labor or poor Apgar scores. Data from the recent Cochrane meta-analysis on use of aspirin for prophylaxis of pre-eclampsia have suggested an overall risk reduction of 15%. However, when aspirin is targeted at women in high-risk groups—for example, when multiple risk factors exist (such as obesity, age, family history)—it may produce a more significant effect. The pregnant obese woman must be screened for fetal anomalies and also for metabolic problems. While hospitalized, thromboprophylaxis is advised in pregnant women who are obese.

Obesity is associated with a higher risk of GDM

Screening for and management of diabetes in pregnancy is important. For those without diabetes, the risk for the fetus of mild hyperglycemia in pregnancy has been underestimated in the past. Even mild hyperglycemia in pregnancy can drive fetal hyperinsulinemia, and this is closely related to the risk of macrosomia and attendant complications. The Hyperglycemia and Adverse Pregnancy Outcomes (HAPO) study has now led to new recommendations for intensive management of this condition.

Surgery for morbid obesity and pregnancy outcomes

An increasing proportion of women in the reproductive age group are morbidly obese and often have other co-morbidities, such as diabetes, hypertension, or sleep apnea. Bariatric surgery is effective in such individuals for weight loss and improving outcomes related to their co-morbidities. A number of women have now had bariatric surgery and subsequently achieved pregnancy, and a number of research papers have sought to quantify the benefits in terms of maternal and fetal clinical outcomes. A systematic review of bariatric surgery and pregnancy outcomes found that gestational diabetes (0% vs 22.1%, $P < 0.05$) and pre-eclampsia (0% vs 3.1%, $P < 0.05$) were lower in the bariatric surgery group compared to morbidly obese women who did not have surgery. Neonatal outcomes such as premature delivery and low birth weight were no different for laparoscopic bands and bypass procedures, whereas the rates of macrosomia were significantly lower (7.7% for surgery vs 14.6% for no surgery, $P < 0.05$). Maternal nutritional deficiencies are a concern, and there is insufficient literature at present on this subject. However, there are a number of case reports of disturbances in coagulation, including neonatal bleeding and intra-uterine death. Deficiencies of iron, calcium, and vitamins B12 and D are also described. This highlights the need for careful management of maternal and fetal nutrition in patients who have had bariatric surgery when they become pregnant.

Reproductive health in men

The prevalence of some degree of erectile dysfunction (ED) in men aged 40–70 years is thought to be about 50%. Symptoms are increased in obese men, and the underlying pathophysiology is believed to be associated with the complications of the metabolic syndrome. In the past decade, ED has become a "hot topic" for developments in medical therapy. However, modifiable health behaviors, including reducing alcohol intake, weight loss, and physical activity, are clearly associated with a reduced risk for ED. Obesity may also affect sperm count and also sperm motility. While the effect on those with morbid obesity is clear, the role of obesity in sub-fertility in those with more modest grades of obesity is less clear and estimates of a threefold increase are quoted with rates approaching around 15% compared to around 5% in normal-weight individuals.

Obesity and reproductive system malignancies

Obesity is a risk factor for endometrial, postmenopausal breast and ovarian cancers in women and prostate cancer in men. In the case of high-grade prostate cancer, obesity appears to be a risk for more aggressive course of the disease. This does not appear to be the case in those with indolent or low-grade tumors. The hormonal milieu in obesity is thought to promote these cancers. Elevated endogenous estrogen levels that persist even after menopause and hyperinsulinemia associated with obesity contribute to carcinogenesis.

Pitfalls

1. Obese women, especially after the mid-30s, seeking treatment for fertility may ignore advice to lose weight because they may feel under pressure to achieve fertility.

2. Patients with PCOS will find it harder to lose weight than those without PCOS. The physician must recognize this and ensure the patient is aware that there are biological reasons for this so they do not perceive this to be entirely their failure.

3. It is important to have the support of the rest of the family when trying to treat the obese woman. Shopping for children or a spouse who insists on energy-dense snacks or old food habits she is trying to change can thwart attempts by health professionals to help produce behavior change in the woman.

4. For those women identified as having gestational diabetes, follow-up is advised periodically after pregnancy, as around 50% will develop T2DM within 5 years.

5. In the obese woman with PCOS, intensive management of obesity is important, as even modest weight loss can restore ovulatory cycles and avoid the need for use of ART.

Key societies

North American Association for Obesity
Association for the Study of Obesity in the UK

Key web links

Institute of Medicine, Report Brief May 2009. Weight gain during pregnancy: re-examining the guidelines. http://www.iom.edu/Reports/2009/Weight-Gain-During-Pregnancy -Reexamining-the-Guidelines.aspx [accessed on December 29, 2012].
http://www.pcosupport.org [accessed on December 29, 2012].
http://www.womenshealth.gov/publications/our-publications/fact-sheet/polycystic-ovary-syndrome.cfm [accessed on December 29, 2012].

Further reading

Barnett, T. & Kumar, S. (2008) Obesity and PCOS. In: *Obesity and Diabetes*, 2nd edn. John Wiley & Sons, Chichester.
Carmichael, A.R. & Bates, T. (2004) Obesity and breast cancer: A review of the literature. *Breast*, 13, 85–92.
Hsing, A.W., Sakoda, L.C., Chua, S., Jr. (2007) Obesity, metabolic syndrome, and prostate cancer. *American Journal of Clinical Nutrition*, 86, s843–s857.
Institute of Medicine, Report Brief May 2009. Weight gain during pregnancy—re-examining the guidelines. http://www.iom.edu/~/media/Files/Report%20Files/2009/Weight-Gain-During-Pregnancy-Reexamining-the-Guidelines/Report%20Brief%20-%20Weight%20Gain%20During%20Pregnancy.pdf [accessed on December 29, 2012].

Maggard, M.A., Yermilov, I., Li, Z. *et al.* (2008) Pregnancy and fertility following bariatric surgery: A systematic review. *Journal of American Medical Association,* 300, 2286–2296.

Metwally, M., Li, T.C. & Ledger, W.L. (2007) The impact of obesity on female reproductive function. *Obesity Reviews,* 8, 515–523.

Modesitt, S.C. & van Nagell, J.R., Jr. (2005) The impact of obesity on the incidence and treatment of gynecologic cancers: A review. *Obstetrical & Gynecological Survey,* 60, 683–692.

Norman, R.J., Noakes, M., Wu, R., Davies, M.J., Mora, L. & Wang, J.X. (2004) Improving reproductive performance in overweight/obese women with effective weight management. *Human Reproduction Update,* 10, 267–280.

Practice Committee of American Society for Reproductive Medicine. (2008) Obesity and reproduction: An educational bulletin. *Fertility and Sterility,* 90 (Suppl.), S21–S29.

Rotterdam ESHRE/ASRM-Sponsored PCOS Consensus Workshop Group. (2004) Revised 2003 consensus on diagnostic criteria and long-term health risks related to polycystic ovary syndrome (PCOS). *Human Reproduction,* 19, 41.

Royal College of Obstetricians and Gynaecologists UK guidelines for the management of women with obesity in pregnancy. http://www.rcog.org.uk/womens-health/clinical-guidance/management-women-obesity-pregnancy [accessed on December 29, 2012].

Tang, T., Lord, J.M., Norman, R.J., Yasmin, E. & Balen, A.H. (2009) Insulin-sensitising drugs (metformin, rosiglitazone, pioglitazone, D-chiro-inositol) for women with polycystic ovary syndrome, oligoamenorrhoea and subfertility. *Cochrane Database of Systematic Reviews,* 4, CD003053.

CHAPTER 15

Gastro-intestinal and Hepatobiliary Disease

Key points

1. Obesity is associated with increased risk of gastritis and reflux esophagitis, gallbladder disease, and NAFLD.
2. GI malignancies are also more common in obesity and must be borne in mind as a cause of unintentional weight loss.
3. NAFLD and esophagitis are improved by weight loss. However, risk of gallstones increases with significant weight loss.
4. The gut is now the focus of many of the newer approaches for the management of obesity. Bariatric surgery can produce some management issues during follow-up, and gut-hormone-based therapies are being developed for medical management of obesity.

CASE STUDIES

Case study 1

LK, a 42-year-old lady with a weight of 250 lb and a BMI of 46 kg/m², had a laparoscopic gastric band operation. She lost 60 lb over 12 months and had been seeing her primary care physician with symptoms of pain in the right upper quadrant. The pain had been getting worse progressively, and she thought it was something to do with her gastric band.

Comment: She consulted her surgeon and an ultrasound scan confirmed gallstones. She subsequently underwent laparoscopic cholecystectomy.

Practical Manual of Clinical Obesity, First Edition. Robert Kushner, Victor Lawrence and Sudhesh Kumar.
© 2013 John Wiley & Sons, Ltd. Published 2013 by John Wiley & Sons, Ltd.

Case study 2

SD, a 40-year-old man with a weight of 250 lb and a BMI of 36 kg/m², was recently diagnosed to have impaired glucose tolerance following an insurance health examination. Liver function tests (LFTs) showed a raised alanine aminotransferase (ALT) of 82 IU, and the liver ultrasound confirmed a fatty liver. He drank about 3–4 units of alcohol a week during weekends, and he was diagnosed to have NAFLD.

Comment: He was given weight loss and lifestyle advice initially with regular exercise and diet, and subsequently he was also treated with orlistat. SD lost over 30 lb over the next year, and LFTs have improved with his ALT now 48 IU. He is very pleased with his progress and continues to maintain his current lifestyle and aims to lose further weight to try and normalize his LFTs.

Case study 3

BR, a 45-year-old male biker, remembers being overweight virtually all his life. He weighed 300 lb and had a BMI of 54 kg/m². He had been attending a weight management clinic since he was told he had high cholesterol at an insurance medical examination. Despite the efforts of the dietician and the psychologist, he did not lose any weight over the following year. However, during a follow-up visit 6 months later, his doctor observed he had lost nearly 30 lb. BR said he had not done anything different but he found it easier to manage his appetite. Four months later he reported some dysphagia and underwent endoscopy. Esophageal carcinoma was diagnosed and scans showed metastasis in the liver. BR died less than a year later.

Comment: The clinician should be alert to the possibility of malignancy as a cause of rapid weight loss in obese individuals as they are at higher risk for certain cancers.

Non-alcoholic fatty liver disease (NAFLD)

NAFLD is one of the most common causes of chronic liver disease globally, mirroring the trends of weight gain and diabetes in developed and developing countries. Non-alcoholic steato-hepatitis (NASH) describes a non-alcohol-related liver disease where histologic features resemble those of alcoholic hepatitis. It is also one of the commonest causes of idiopathic cirrhosis today. It is estimated that roughly 20–30% of the adult population in many developed countries have NAFLD and 1–3% have NASH. The key features are hepatic steatosis, where liver fat is in excess of 10% of total weight, and also evidence of elevated liver transaminases where the pattern is that ALT is typically higher than aspartate aminotransferase (AST). NASH is also a risk factor for diabetes.

Natural history of NAFLD

Long-term outcomes in NAFLD can vary considerably. Simple steatosis is typically benign and stable with a 1–2% risk of developing clinical evidence of cirrhosis over 15–20 years. At the other end of the spectrum, patients with NASH are at an increased risk for developing cirrhosis, end-stage liver failure, and hepatocellular carcinoma. However, the risk of progression to cirrhosis or hepatocellular carcinoma is low and is around 3% and 15% over 10 and 20 years, respectively. Nevertheless, because of the large numbers of people affected, this is now a significant cause of both cirrhosis and hepatocellular carcinoma worldwide.

NAFLD and diabetes

Epidemiological studies confirm the association between NAFLD and diabetes. The liver has an important contribution to make in insulin resistance, and conversely insulin resistance aggravates the biochemical processes that lead to NASH. Elevated serum insulin that is secondary to insulin resistance in respect to carbohydrate metabolism drives lipogenesis and promotes steatosis in the liver. The enzymes related to lipogenesis in the liver remain insulin sensitive in the obese. It is thought that reactive oxidant stress and inflammation followed by fibrosis provide the second "hit" after fatty liver for the development of NASH. Diabetes is associated with increased oxidant stress and thus may increase risk of NASH on a background of fatty liver.

Diagnosis of NAFLD

A definitive diagnosis of NAFLD requires exclusion of alcohol abuse and histologic confirmation, although performing a liver biopsy in all patients with suspected steatosis is not practical. The precise level of daily ethanol intake that conclusively distinguishes non-alcoholic from alcoholic disease is not known. The NIH Clinical Research Network on NAFLD has reached a consensus that defines that the maximum allowed alcohol intake level for NAFLD diagnosis is 140 g ethanol/week (two standard drinks per day) for men and 70 g ethanol/week (one standard drink per day) for women. Detailed information concerning previous alcohol habits should also be obtained, since the overall lifetime consumption appears to be significant.

The need to perform a liver biopsy to establish the diagnosis is still debated due to the risk of complications and limitations associated with sampling and interpretation errors. Nevertheless, histologic assessment is considered important in managing patients with high clinical suspicion for NASH, since the underlying type and stage of NAFLD determine the prognosis and therapeutic strategy. Clinical and laboratory predictors of underlying severity have been reported in order to support a justified selection of the NAFLD patients who would benefit most from a biopsy, but their accuracy to predict more advanced histology is not known.

The diagnosis is suspected by exclusion of alcohol abuse, and ideally a liver biopsy is necessary to be certain but is often not practical. The presence of steatosis and the typical pattern of LFT results together with the exclusion of viral hepatitis and autoimmune or congenital liver diseases usually make NASH the most likely diagnosis. This also involves checking serum ferritin, ceruloplasmin, auto-antibodies, and alpha-1 antitrypsin. New bio-marker-based tests are currently being investigated and include the enhanced liver fibrosis (ELF) test. The key points for the diagnosis of NAFLD are summarized in Table 15.1.

Managing the obese patient with NAFLD

Specific treatment guidelines for NAFLD are lacking because of the paucity of appropriate trials of treatments. Weight loss remains the only established treatment for NAFLD. The presence of abnormal LFTs is often a factor that may motivate patients to achieve weight loss. Monounsaturated fat diets have been shown to reduce liver fat, but large-scale trials with sufficient follow-up are lacking. Co-existing metabolic disorders such as diabetes should be looked for and managed. These patients should restrict or even abstain from alcohol consumption after the diagnosis of NAFLD in order to avoid additional stress to the liver. Aiming for 10% weight loss through diet and regular exercise is recommended in these patients, and referral to a dietician may be helpful.

There is no specific drug therapy for NAFLD. Metformin has initially yielded contradictory results regarding long-term improvement in biochemical and histologic features of NAFLD. Recent data are more supportive of the effects of metformin in reducing steatosis, hepatic cellular

Table 15.1 Key points in the diagnostic process for NAFLD.

Definite diagnosis	Symptoms and signs	Laboratory	Imaging
Alcohol	Asymptomatic (50–100%)	↑ ALT, AST	Ultrasonography
Men <2 standard drinks/day	Fatigue (0–70%) RUQ pain (0–50%)	Usually ALT, AST <2–4× upper normal	Computed tomography (CT) Magnetic resonance imaging (MRI)
Women <1 standard drink/day	Hepatomegaly Splenomegaly (rare)	Usually ALT > AST ↑ ALP, GGT ↑ IgA (about 25%)	Magnetic resonance spectroscopy Reliable for diagnosis
Liver biopsy Histologic confirmation and staging	Palmar erythema (rare)	Hyperglycemia (about 30–35%) Hyperlipidemia (about 20–30%)	Not reliable for staging

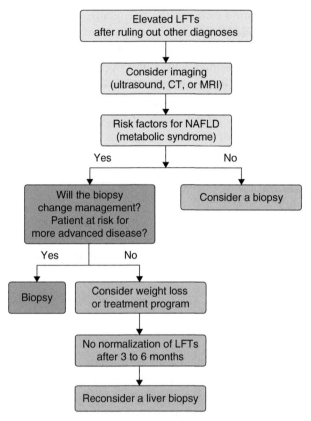

Figure 15.1 Flow chart for diagnosis of NAFLD. Reproduced from http://www.clevelandclinicmeded.com/medicalpubs/diseasemanagement/hepatology/nonalcoholic-fatty-liver-disease/

injury, and inflammation. Liver transplantation represents the last option in the treatment of NASH-related cirrhosis. Notably, many of these patients are also expected to be poor candidates for transplantation due to severe co-morbidities. Thus, prevention and early intervention are regarded as vital in NAFLD patients (Figure 15.1).

Gallbladder disease

Obesity is associated with increased gallbladder disease in those aged over 60 years. The most common problem is related to gallstones. Obesity is characterized by a high daily cholesterol turnover, which is proportional to the total body fat mass and can result in elevated biliary cholesterol secretion. The resultant supersaturation of the bile then makes it more lithogenic with high cholesterol concentrations relative to bile acids and phospholipids. Around 10–15% of men and 20–40% of women have gallstones on ultrasound examination. Generally, women have a higher prevalence of gallstones than men. In the Nurses' Health Study, women with a BMI over 30 kg/m² had twice the risk of gallstones compared to non-obese women and women with a BMI over 45 kg/m² had a sevenfold higher risk compared to those with a BMI less than 24 kg/m².

Although weight loss is generally beneficial for most diseases associated with obesity, in the case of gallstones, the opposite is true. Weight loss either through dieting or bariatric surgery is associated with a further increase in the incidence of gallstone formation. The clinician should therefore have a high index of suspicion for gallstones in obese individuals especially over the age of 45 years. They are readily dealt with by laparoscopic surgery.

Obesity is also associated with an increased risk of gallbladder cancer, attributed to higher risk of cholelithiasis and chronic inflammation. This is a rare type of cancer but is becoming more of a problem with the growing epidemic of obesity.

Gastritis and GERD

Increase in the prevalence of obesity worldwide is associated with an increase in the prevalence of GERD. Obesity has been shown in several epidemiological studies to have a causal effect on GERD symptoms, erosive symptoms, and esophageal carcinoma. The increase in intragastric pressure, gastroesophageal gradient, transient lower esophageal sphincter relaxations, and esophageal acid exposure appears to be a contributory factor. Other contributing factors are esophagogastric junction incompetence and esophageal clearance mechanisms. Aging population and decrease in the prevalence of *Helicobacter* infection are also factors responsible for increase in the prevalence of GERD. Symptoms of GERD seem to be more severe and more resistant to treatment with proton pump inhibitors in patients with obesity.

Obese individuals have greater volumes of gastric fluid and increased intra-abdominal pressure, which predisposes to a higher risk of aspiration. Patients reporting chronic cough may be experiencing micro-aspiration at night.

Managing the obese patient with GERD

Weight loss is the most important and effective management of GERD in patients with obesity. Consumption of smaller food portions and reducing the consumption of alcohol and greasy foods may help. In the short term, it may be necessary to treat symptoms with proton pump inhibitors, but these are less effective than in subjects without obesity who have GERD. Bariatric surgery usually results in significant weight loss and also causes resolution or significant reduction of symptoms of GERD. Gastric bypass reduces the volume of gastric acid secretion in the stomach near the esophagus and so is more effective. If there is insignificant weight loss with a gastric band, and if the band is tightened too much, then this can lead to worsening of symptoms. Some patients may require surgery for reflux esophagitis (Nissen fundoplication), and this may be combined with a gastric bypass operation. Weight loss is key for the improvement or resolution of symptoms of GERD.

Other GI disorders

Functional bowel disorders and GI malignancies are increased in obesity. The latter must be borne in mind when rapid weight loss is seen in someone who has normally struggled to lose weight. Recently, there is considerable interest in gut microbiota and its alteration in obese individuals. These changes could have implications for metabolic and immune functions, but it is not clear if the differences observed are the result or the cause of obesity. There are claims that probiotics produce a number of health benefits, including weight loss and functional improvements in the bowel, but these claims have not been evaluated in randomized controlled clinical trials to provide robust evidence at this time. This is an area that is currently a subject of further research.

Pitfalls

1. Statins are not contra-indicated in patients with NAFLD/NASH, and liver function may actually improve following treatment of dyslipidemia.
2. Consider other causes of liver dysfunction in the obese, as viral hepatitis, alcoholic or drug-induced liver disease, and undiagnosed inherited disorders may also co-exist. When in doubt, refer to a gastroenterologist especially if liver function does not appear to improve despite weight loss.
3. GI malignancies are more common in people with obesity. Beware of assuming that weight loss is always intentional especially when the patient has previously not managed lifestyle modification successfully.
4. Individuals with obesity may underreport the amount of alcohol being consumed. Seeing the patient with other family members can reveal inconsistencies in reported intake.

Key web links

American College of Gastroenterology Toolkit for Physicians on Obesity and Gastrointestinal Disease.   http://d2j7fjepcxuj0a.cloudfront.net/wp-content/uploads/2011/07/institute-ACG_Obesity_Physician_Resource_Guide.pdf [accessed on December 29, 2012].
http://www.digestive.niddk.nih.gov/ddiseases/pubs/nash/ [accessed on December 29, 2012].

Further reading

Anand, G. & Katz, P.O. (2010) Gastroesophageal reflux disease and obesity. *Gastroenterology Clinics of North America*, 39, 39–46.

Balaban, Y.H. (2011) A key problem and challenge for hepatology: Obesity-related metabolic liver diseases. *World Journal of Hepatology*, 3, 142–146.

Chen, Y., Wang, X., Wang, J., Yan, Z. & Luo, J. (2012) Excess body weight and the risk of primary liver cancer: An updated meta-analysis of prospective studies. *European Journal of Cancer*, 48, 2137–2145.

Fabbrini, E., Sullivan, S. & Klein, S. (2010) Obesity and nonalcoholic fatty liver disease: Biochemical, metabolic, and clinical implications. *Hepatology*, 51, 679–689.

Festi, D., Schiumerini, R., Birtolo, C. *et al.* (2011) Gut microbiota and its pathophysiology in disease paradigms. *Digestive Diseases*, 29, 518–524.

Ho, W. & Spiegel, B.M. (2008) The relationship between obesity and functional gastrointestinal disorders: Causation, association, or neither? *Gastroenterology Hepatology*, 4, 572–578.

Hong, S., Cai, Q., Chen, D., Zhu, W., Huang, W. & Li, Z. (2012) Abdominal obesity and the risk of colorectal adenoma: A meta-analysis of observational studies. *European Journal of Cancer Prevention*, 21, 523–531.

Lagergren, J. (2011) Influence of obesity on the risk of esophageal disorders. *Nature Reviews Gastroenterology & Hepatology*, 8, 340–347.

Maclure, K.M., Hayes, K.C., Colditz, G.A., Stampfer, M.J., Speizer, F.E. & Willett, W.C. (1989) Weight, diet, and the risk of symptomatic gallstones in middle-aged women. *New England Journal of Medicine*, 321, 563–569.

Madalosso, C.A., Gurski, R.R., Callegari-Jacques, S.M., Navarini, D., Thiesen, V. & Fornari, F. (2010) The impact of gastric bypass on gastroesophageal reflux disease in patients with morbid obesity: A prospective study based on the Montreal Consensus. *Annals of Surgery*, 251, 244–248.

CHAPTER 16

Respiratory Disease

Key points

- Obesity is associated with myriad abnormalities in pulmonary function, but most significantly, it increases the risk of obstructive sleep apnea (OSA).
- In obese patients with OSA, it is often also associated with other cardiovascular risk factors, such as hypertension, dyslipidemia, and diabetes.
- Treatment of OSA can bring about many benefits, including better engagement with lifestyle behavior change and also reduction in blood pressure.
- Weight loss can improve symptoms of OSA, and with major weight loss, OSA may disappear.

CASE STUDIES

Case study 1

AA, a 42-year-old bank executive, was getting concerned about his poor memory. He used to be regarded as somewhat of a "whizz kid." He was concerned at the rate at which he was having difficulty with his memory, and this was affecting his work. He also noticed that he often nodded off to sleep at meetings especially in the afternoon after lunch. One evening he had fallen asleep while the car was stationary in a traffic jam, which prompted a visit to the doctor. He weighed 270 lb and his BMI was 42 kg/m², and his collar size was 19. His blood pressure was 180/95 mmHg, and he was also found to have a cholesterol level of 6.4 mmol/L.

Comment: He scored 12 on the Epworth Sleepiness Scale questionnaire and he was referred to a respiratory physician who arranged overnight polysomnography, which confirmed sleep apnea. He was subsequently put on continuous positive airway pressure (CPAP), and he soon felt much better. When reviewed 2 months later, he no longer had problems with daytime sleepiness or memory problems.

Case study 2

AB, a 35-year-old computer programmer, had been putting on weight rapidly over the years. He was aware that junk food and cola coupled with a lack of exercise and drinking

---

Practical Manual of Clinical Obesity, First Edition. Robert Kushner, Victor Lawrence and Sudhesh Kumar.
© 2013 John Wiley & Sons, Ltd. Published 2013 by John Wiley & Sons, Ltd.

beer on most nights was to blame. He weighed 360 lb and had a BMI of 55 kg/m² with severe OSA, and he had been given a CPAP mask to help treat his OSA. However, he hardly used it because it was uncomfortable and he could not sleep with it at night. As a result, he was very sleepy during the day and was often found by co-workers asleep at his computer table. When he fell asleep during an important meeting and snored loudly, his boss made it clear he had to do something about it. He attempted weight loss by himself and also tried various diets. He had only managed to lose 2 lb over the last 6 months and was very frustrated that he was unable to lose weight, although he appreciated that this would improve his symptoms of OSA.

Comment: He was referred for a gastric band and lost 40 lb in 6 months, and he no longer felt sleepy during the day. He felt that he had much more energy, and he had no OSA on repeat polysomnography. It also transformed his performance at work.

Obesity and lung function

Obesity produces a restrictive ventilatory defect that increases with obesity but also results in a decrease in various parameters of lung function, including total lung capacity, forced expiratory volume in one second (FEV1), forced vital capacity (FVC), functional residual capacity, and expiratory reserve volume. It is mainly due to the respiratory system having to work harder to eliminate CO_2 because of the increased body weight and visceral adiposity preventing proper movement of the diaphragm. Studies also demonstrate inefficiencies in gas exchange in individuals with obesity. Therefore, individuals with obesity have a combination of reduced distensibility of the thorax, reduced diaphragm movement, increased ventilatory effort, and reduced gas exchange, which all adversely affect lung function and worsen symptoms of pre-existing lung conditions like asthma and chronic obstructive airway disease (COPD). Needless to say, smoking compounds all of these problems. Also, physical activity results in a greater metabolic stress during exercise in individuals with obesity.

Common respiratory diseases associated with obesity

The most common obesity-related respiratory disorder is sleep-disordered breathing, also called obstructive sleep apnea (OSA). This is discussed in detail later in this chapter. Reversible obstructive airway disease and COPD both appear to be common in obese individuals. Asthma and obesity have been shown to be associated epidemiologically. The relative risk varies between 1.4- and 2.2-fold, depending on the population studied, with a clear increasing risk noted with increasing BMI. A causal relationship has not been clearly established, although factors associated with one can be linked as risk factors for the other. For example, reduced physical activity or steroid treatment common in asthma is a risk for obesity, and the pro-inflammatory hormonal and cytokine milieu or the observation of greater bronchial hyper-reactivity in an obese individual is a risk factor for asthma.

When asthma or COPD is present with obesity, there is a definite negative effect of obesity on the asthma- or COPD-related health. Treatment of the reversible obstructive airway disease with inhaled steroids is often unavoidable, and severe asthma attacks or associated chest infections require oral steroid therapy, which is associated with further weight gain. Every effort must be made to avoid acute exacerbations of COPD or asthma, and avoidance of allergens may reduce the requirement for steroids. Weight loss results in improvement of respiratory symptoms, and weight loss through lifestyle measures including diet and physical activity should be encouraged. Where appropriate, weight loss medication can be prescribed, and bariatric surgery has been shown to improve respiratory prognosis through weight loss.

Obstructive sleep apnea (OSA)

Obstructive sleep apnea (OSA) is part of a spectrum of sleep-disordered breathing syndromes that range from heavy snoring to profound nocturnal hypoventilation and respiratory failure during sleep. Simple snoring is not considered part of this syndrome. OSA is characterized by repetitive episodes of complete cessation of airflow (apnea) or measurable reduction in airflow (hypopnea) during sleep due to collapse of the upper airway, generally at the level of the pharynx. During an apnea, continued respiratory efforts occur against the closed airway, with resulting hypoxemia, until the apnea is terminated by arousal from sleep with restoration of upper airway patency. Typically, after a few deep breaths, this cycle is repeated, often hundreds of times through the night. The recurrent arousals cause sleep fragmentation resulting in daytime sleepiness, and most of the time, the patient is not aware of these short recurrent arousals.

Obesity, especially central obesity, is one of the strongest risk factors for OSA, and external neck circumference is an index of neck fat deposition, particularly in the lateral pharyngeal fat pads, and may lead to airway narrowing. Neck circumference is increased in patients with OSA and may explain some of the link between obesity and OSA. While OSA is an associated co-morbidity with obesity, there are other sleep-related disorders with obesity. These include inadequate sleep due to lifestyle or insomnia, shift work, depression, intake of alcohol or medications like benzodiazepines and beta-blockers, narcolepsy, idiopathic hypersomnolence syndrome, or periodic leg movement disorder.

Population studies show that the prevalence of OSA with daytime sleepiness is approximately 3–7% for adult males and 2–5% for adult females in the general population. Increasing BMI is known to increase the prevalence of OSA, and weight gain over time is known to increase OSA, with 10% weight gain resulting in increase of apnea–hypopnea index (AHI) by 32%. Increasing age increases the risk of OSA until it reaches a plateau at age 60. Men are four times more likely to have OSA compared to women. Familial clustering of OSA has been noted, independent of age and obesity. OSA is more common in certain genetic syndromes, like Pierre Robin syndrome, Down syndrome, and Marfan syndrome. Certain endocrine abnormalities are also associated with OSA, including hypothyroidism, acromegaly, and Cushing syndrome.

Symptoms and signs of OSA

History and physical examination have fairly poor sensitivity and specificity for the detection of sleep-disordered breathing. The typical symptoms associated with OSA are heavy snoring and excessive daytime sleepiness. The reporting of witnessed apneas is a relatively specific symptom but is also relatively insensitive. Other symptoms are listed in Table 16.1.

Diagnosis and severity of OSA

Sleep-disordered breathing should be considered an important co-morbidity of obesity that improves with weight loss, and there must be a high index of suspicion in individuals with obesity. The two commonly used questionnaire-based tools to screen for possible sleep apnea are the Epworth Sleepiness Scale (Table 16.2) and the Berlin questionnaire. Those with a high score in these must be referred for polysomnography to confirm the diagnosis. However,

Table 16.1 Common symptoms associated with OSA.

Snoring
Daytime sleepiness
Disrupted sleep
Choking or gasping during sleep
Dry throat/mouth in the morning
Morning headaches
Nocturia
Heartburn
Poor memory/concentration
Fatigue
Impotence
Altered mood/irritability

Table 16.2 Epworth Sleepiness Scale.

Situation	Chance of dozing
Refers to your usual way of life in recent times. Even if you have not done some of these things recently, try to work out how they would have affected you.	0 = would never doze 1 = slight chance of dozing 2 = moderate chance of dozing 3 = high chance of dozing
Sitting and reading Watching TV Sitting, inactive, in a public place As a passenger in a car for an hour Lying down in the afternoon Sitting and talking to someone Sitting quietly after a lunch without alcohol In a car, while stopped for a few minutes in traffic **Total**[a]	

Reproduced from Johns *Sleep* 1991; 14:540–545.
Scores of 10 or more suggest excessive daytime somnolence and warrant referral to a specialist for further investigations.

these questionnaires are not 100% sensitive or specific, so if there is a strong clinical suspicion, patients should still be referred for further assessment.

The "gold standard" approach to the investigation of sleep-disordered breathing is an overnight in-laboratory sleep study (polysomnography). The expense and inconvenience of polysomnography have led to a search for alternative tools for the diagnosis of OSA, which now include overnight oximetry and portable or "at-home" systems. They can detect repetitive oxygen desaturations seen in OSA and can be diagnostic in some patients, but a normal study does not exclude OSA. AHI is the number of episodes of apnea or hypopnea per hour. According to the American Academy of Sleep Medicine, an AHI of less than 5 is normal, 5–15 is mild OSA, 15–30 is moderate OSA, and more than 30 is severe OSA.

Consequences of OSA

Excessive daytime sleepiness is characteristic of OSA, and people with OSA perform poorly on psychometric tests compared to controls. Sleep apnea leads to defects in executive function and working memory in both adults and children, and data from the SOS study show that, in equally obese men and women, OSA is associated with impaired work performance, increased sick leave, and a higher divorce rate.

Cardiovascular consequences of OSA are significant, and acute effects are an increase in systemic and pulmonary blood pressure along with nocturnal hypoxia and rise in sympathetic nerve activity. Chronic systemic hypertension is strongly associated with obesity, and treatment of OSA with CPAP results in a reduction in blood pressure. Causal data for OSA as a cause of hypertension are hard to obtain as there are a large number of major confounders including obesity and age, although data from two large studies, the Sleep Heart Health Study and Wisconsin Sleep Cohort Study, have shown OSA to be a risk factor for hypertension independent of obesity. There is a large body of evidence linking OSA to cardiovascular events and mortality, but causality again is difficult to prove due to associated hypertension, obesity, and age.

OSA has been linked to impaired glucose tolerance, insulin resistance, and T2DM. This cluster of risk factors has been referred to as "syndrome Z." This association remains independent of obesity, although improvement in these parameters following treatment of OSA with CPAP remains a topic of debate. Men with OSA have a defect in both growth hormone and testosterone secretion independent of obesity, and this improves with CPAP treatment without weight change.

Nocturnal pulmonary hypertension is present in OSA early in the course of the disease. However, daytime pulmonary hypertension is seen in 10–40% of patients with OSA even after exclusion of other lung diseases. Long-standing OSA can lead to obesity hypoventilation syndrome (OHS), discussed next.

Obesity hypoventilation syndrome (OHS)

The majority of patients with OSA have normal arterial carbon dioxide tensions ($PaCO_2$) when awake. The term obesity hypoventilation syndrome (OHS) describes those patients with obesity and daytime respiratory failure (hypercapnia and usually also hypoxemia) in the absence of lung or neuromuscular disease. It is likely that the development of OHS is multifactorial, with the key elements a combination of obesity (increased upper airway loading and reduced lung volumes), OSA, poor chemoreceptor function (particularly defective arousal responses to hypoxia), and possibly alcohol consumption (reducing upper airway tone and arousal responses to asphyxia).

Upper airway obstruction is a crucial factor in the pathogenesis of OHS, and relief of upper airway obstruction by tracheostomy effectively treats the respiratory failure.

Management algorithm for OSA

Weight loss is the most important treatment for OSA. Even a moderate weight loss of 10% body weight results in the reduction of AHI of 26–50%.

The morbidly obese patient with sleep apnea may require bariatric surgery if medical weight management does not produce clinically meaningful weight loss, with a recent meta-analysis showing dramatic improvements in OSA after surgery and an 85.7% resolution of OSA. Therefore, patients with OSA and a BMI greater than $40\,kg/m^2$ should be a priority for bariatric surgery.

In addition to weight loss, general advice to improve symptoms of OSA should include avoidance of alcohol and benzodiazepines. These can reduce pharyngeal muscle tone and depress arousal responses, resulting in more and longer apneas during sleep. Similarly, sleep deprivation can impair upper airway muscle tone and increase arousal thresholds, increasing any tendency to OSA. Smoking cessation can reduce self-reported snoring, possibly by effects of smoke on airway inflammation, and should be encouraged.

Sleep apnea is readily treatable with CPAP, which involves the patient sleeping with a tight mask on their face. Many patients find this a little awkward at first, but there are many machines available, and different sized masks, so there is a good chance that one of them will suit the patient. However, some still struggle and do not use the machine often enough. Mandibular advancement devices (MADs) are intraoral ortho-dontic devices designed to displace the mandible anteriorly, increasing the anteroposterior diameter of the upper airway and so reducing upper airway closure and collapse when worn at night. These devices are effective in reducing snoring, assessed both objectively and subjectively, but the effects of these devices in OSA are less clear and are not as definite as those noted with CPAP. The American Academy of Sleep Medicine's clinical practice guidelines for the treatment of snoring and OSA state that MADs are now indicated for mild to moderate OSA in patients who prefer oral appliances to CPAP, who do not respond to or are not suitable for treatment with CPAP, or in whom treatment attempts with CPAP are unsuccessful. CPAP should be considered before oral appliances in severe OSA and those in whom urgent treatment is required to treat severe symptoms (e.g., sleepiness) or significant co-morbidities (e.g., cardiovascular). MAD patients require sufficient teeth to retain the device. Caution is needed for those with periodontal dis-ease or temporomandibular disease. External nasal dilator strips may help with snoring but have no effect on OSA.

Reduced concentration and tiredness, along with daytime somnolence, result in patients with OSA being less receptive to weight loss advice. Successful treatment of sleep apnea makes the patient less sleepy and more alert, and often then it is a good time to engage the patient more effectively in weight loss.

> **Pitfalls**
> 1. Do not assume that all patients with OSA will get better with CPAP, as many patients do not tolerate the mask.
> 2. In a patient with a convincing history, consider polysomnography despite a negative Epworth Sleepiness Scale score, as patients may underreport sleepiness, especially in relation to driving for fear of losing their license.
> 3. Although OSA may be the most common cause, do not ignore other causes of sleepiness in the obese.
> 4. Do not forget to counsel against drinking alcohol in excess.
> 5. Patients with obesity and sleep apnea also often have other cardiovascular risk factors, such as diabetes, hypertension, and dyslipidemia, which should not be missed.

Key web links

American Academy of Sleep Medicine. http://www.aasmnet.org/ [accessed on December 29, 2012].

British Sleep Society. http://www.sleeping.org.uk/ [accessed on December 29, 2012].

European Sleep Research Society. http://www.esrs.eu/ [accessed on December 29, 2012].

Further reading

American Academy of Sleep Medicine. (2005) *International Classification of Sleep Disorders: Diagnostic and Coding Manual*, 2nd ed. American Academy of Sleep Medicine, Westchester.

Crummy, F., Piper, A.J. & Naughton, M.T. (2008) Obesity and the lung: 2. Obesity and sleep-disordered breathing. *Thorax*, 63, 738–746.

Lugogo, N.L., Kraft, M. & Dixon, A.E. (2010) Does obesity produce a distinct asthma phenotype? *Journal of Applied Physiology*, 108, 729–734.

Netzer, N.C., Stoohs, R.A., Netzer, C.M., Clark, K. & Strohl, K.P. (1999) Using the Berlin Questionnaire to identify patients at risk for the sleep apnea syndrome. *Annals of Internal Medicine*, 131, 485–491.

Pannain, S. & Mokhlesi, B. (2010) Bariatric surgery and its impact on sleep architecture, sleep-disordered breathing, and metabolism. *Best Practice & Research. Clinical Endocrinology & Metabolism*, 24, 745–761.

Salome, C.M., King, G.G. & Berend, N. (2010) Physiology of obesity and effects on lung function. *Journal of Applied Physiology*, 108, 206–211.

Simard, B., Turcotte, H., Marceau, P., *et al.* Asthma and sleep apnea in patients with morbid obesity: Outcome after bariatric surgery. *Obesity Surgery*, 14, 1381–1388.

Zammit, C., Liddicoat, H., Moonsie, I. & Makker, H. (2010) Obesity and respiratory diseases. *International Journal of General Medicine*, 3, 335–343.

CHAPTER 17

Obesity and Cardiovascular Disease

Key points

1. Obesity is associated with hypertension, dyslipidemia, and diabetes, all of which are cardiovascular risk factors. Although obesity clusters with these risk factors, it also has its own independent and additional effect on the risk of cardiovascular events including myocardial infarction and stroke.

2. Central rather than gluteo-femoral adiposity confers greater vascular risk for any given BMI. Central fat distribution is a risk factor for vascular events even in normal-weight individuals.

3. The atherogenic lipid profile in obesity is not simply due to raised serum cholesterol but also due to high levels of highly atherogenic, small, dense LDL, low levels of HDL, and raised serum triglyceride.

4. Obesity and metabolic syndrome are also associated with sleep apnea. Diagnosis and treatment of sleep apnea can result in successful control of previously refractory hypertension.

5. "Fitness" and "fatness" are both very important modifiable risk factors for vascular disease. However, fitness improves (perhaps halves) but does not completely abolish the cardiovascular risk of fatness.

6. The concept of "syndrome Z" has been advanced to describe the combination of the metabolic "syndrome X" with OSA. This is a particularly dangerous combination creating a "perfect storm" of hypertension, sympathetic activation, and obesity-related cardiomyopathy superimposed on a background of increased atherosclerotic risk and a pro-coagulant state.

Practical Manual of Clinical Obesity, First Edition. Robert Kushner, Victor Lawrence and Sudhesh Kumar.

CASE STUDIES

Case study 1

AW, a 62-year-old man, attended hospital with a new onset of central chest pain, which developed after running to catch an elevator. He smoked cigarettes, had a BMI of 55 kg/m², high blood pressure of 180/100 mmHg, and attributed his gradually progressive weight gain to his job as a telephone operator in the local hospital. Biochemistry results showed a total cholesterol of 240 mg/dL with a low HDL cholesterol of 36 mg/dL. He also had a fasting glucose of 6.5 mmol/L.

Comment: A diagnosis of non-ST elevation myocardial infarction was made on the basis of abnormal troponin I testing. Coronary angiography was not feasible at the local referral center due to his body habitus, and he was therefore treated medically in the first instance. His cardiovascular risk was reduced significantly by prescription of a statin agent for his dyslipidemia, angiotensin-converting-enzyme inhibitor, antiplatelet agents including aspirin and clopidogrel, and a beta-blocker. OSA was considered, and after a strongly positive Epworth Sleepiness Score, he underwent an overnight polysomnography test and was treated with nasal CPAP at night. He was assessed by the cardiac rehabilitation team and a graded exercise program devised. Review of his diet by a nutritionist was undertaken and significant changes recommended.

Although he did not have invasive coronary intervention, his risk of further coronary events was significantly reduced and many treatable aspects of his obesity belatedly recognized. He aimed in the first instance to avoid the development of T2DM through increased physical activity and mildly hypocaloric diet. His primary physician will consider addition of metformin to his medication depending on the results of repeat fasting blood glucose analysis.

Case study 2

TW, a 55-year-old forklift driver, was popular in his local community for being jolly and friendly. He used to enjoy eating out and was apparently healthy despite weighing over 300 lb and smoking cigars regularly. He made light of advice to lose weight or stop smoking from his doctor and even his friends who would often comment on his legendary snoring. He had felt reassured by a visit to the doctor 3 years ago when he was told his cholesterol was only mildly elevated and he did not have diabetes. He did not consider himself to have hypertension despite mildly elevated readings on most occasions when he visited the doctor, which he attributed to the stress of the visit.

Comment: One day he did not turn up to work, and he was later discovered in bed, dead. An autopsy did not reveal a myocardial infarction, and the most likely cause was considered to be an arrhythmia causing sudden cardiac arrest.

Introduction

Obesity is a risk factor for CVD via its association with insulin resistance, hyperinsulinemia, T2DM, hypertension, and dyslipidemia.

However, the effect of obesity on most vascular outcome measures is not entirely removed after adjustment for these known risk factors, suggesting that obesity has an independent effect which is additive to that of these known vascular risk factors. This effect may be partially explained by the pro-inflammatory and pro-coagulant effects of visceral obesity but may also derive from sympathetic nervous system (SNS) activation and the cardiovascular consequences of OSA syndrome, which becomes increasingly prevalent with advancing obesity (approximately 2–4% in the non-obese and 40% or more in those falling under class III obesity).

The epithet "syndrome Z" has been advanced to describe the particularly dangerous combination of the metabolic "syndrome X" with OSA.

Obesity and CVD risk

Obesity increases the risk of vascular disease, both coronary heart disease and peripheral vascular disease. Obesity is often associated with other metabolic risk factors for vascular disease including T2DM, hypertension, and hyperlipidemia. Although increasing BMI correlates positively with the risk of vascular disease, the degree of abdominal adiposity (assessed using waist circumference, waist–hip ratio (WHR), or DEXA scans) appears to confer the greatest risk. Despite this, BMI remains the most commonly used measure because it is easier to perform, has no cost implications, and is suitable for use in larger epidemiological studies as well as in routine clinical practice.

There is epidemiological evidence of an incremental increase in all-cause mortality with increasing BMI (Figure 17.1). In prospective studies in the National Cancer Institute Cohort Consortium of 1.46 million White adults, overweight and obesity are associated with increased all-cause mortality compared to the lowest mortality with a BMI of 20–24.9 kg/m². In the Prospective Studies Collaboration of 900,000 adults (mostly in western Europe and North America), BMI was a strong predictor of overall mortality with the apparent optimum of about 22.5–25.0 kg/m². The effects of obesity, and particularly fat distribution, on coronary heart disease risk have also been shown to occur in both men and women. Over 11 years, a study of Finnish men showed that a WHR of 0.91 increased the risk of coronary events by almost threefold. In an 8-year follow-up of the US Nurses' Health Study, waist circumference and WHR were strongly and independently associated with an increased age-adjusted risk of coronary heart disease among women.

The adverse effects of abdominal fat distribution may even be seen in relatively lean individuals (BMI < 25 kg/m²). For example, after adjusting for BMI and other cardiac risk factors, women with a WHR of 0.88 or higher had a relative risk of coronary heart disease of 3.25, as compared with those with a WHR below 0.72, and similar findings have been

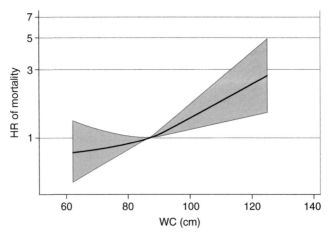

Figure 17.1 Hazard ratios (HRs) and 95% confidence intervals of mortality according to waist circumference (WC) in 1993–1997 with adjustments for BMI. Reproduced from Berentzen *et al.* [1], with permission from the Public Library of Science.

reported in men. Abdominal obesity and waist circumference are especially relevant in non-White populations such as those of South Asian descent where BMI tends to underestimate the degree of abdominal obesity.

Not only is the risk of experiencing a vascular event increased by obesity, particularly central obesity, but the consequences of vascular athero-sclerotic plaque rupture may be magnified by the prothrombotic and inflammatory metabolic profile that accompanies visceral obesity. Treatment options may occasionally be restricted by extreme degrees of obesity result-ing in unfavorable outcomes.

Physical fitness and cardiovascular risk in obesity

Lack of physical fitness is a well-known risk factor for CVD and is statistically associated with obesity. There has been considerable public and professional interest in the "fit–fat" concept, that is, improvement of cardiovascular risk by focusing on healthy lifestyle (fitness) as a primary goal rather than as a means toward achieving weight loss.

Current evidence suggests that physical fitness may reduce the excess cardiovascular mortality risk of obesity by up to a half, but it does not appear to be able to abolish it altogether. Clearly, pursuing increased physical fitness is an important component of any obesity management plan, and its many other benefits (e.g., in maintaining weight lost, avoid-ing diabetes, and improving general well-being) make it a helpful strategy regardless of its efficacy in preventing CVD.

Obesity and hypertension

Obesity is associated with high blood pressure, and weight loss results in an improvement in blood pressure as well as regression of some of its effects on the heart and circulation. The precise pathophysiology causing hypertension in obesity is not currently fully understood but it probably involves increases in cardiac output and total peripheral resistance mediated by a combination of increased SNS activity, hyperinsulinemia, and activation of the renin–angiotensin system. Increased intra-abdominal pressure in those with central obesity may further elevate both systolic and diastolic blood pressures. The characteristic hypertension of obesity tends to be salt sensitive and is frequently more difficult to manage than hypertension in lean individuals, often requiring several agents. It is important to use an appropriately sized cuff for diagnosis and management. as inappropriately small (narrow) cuffs used in an obese individual will spuriously overestimate blood pressure.

Activation of the SNS occurs early in obesity and is involved in many of its chronic manifestations including hypertension, left ventricular hypertrophy, CHF, and arrhythmias. CHF and end-stage renal failure are major complications of chronic essential hypertension in obesity, especially where complicated by T2DM. Despite these observations, there are currently no specific guidelines on the management of obesity-induced hypertension, and although the possibility of using vasodilating beta-blockers in combination with inhibitors of the renin–angiotensin system is theoretically appealing, current data are not sufficient to recommend this yet for general use.

Obesity and stroke

Obesity is associated with an increased risk of stroke even after controlling for its associations with known stroke risk factors, including hypertension, diabetes, and hyperlipidemia. Obesity *per se* is therefore an independent stroke risk factor. In one study, the risk of stroke, after controlling for other risk factors, increased by around 6% for each BMI unit over $25\,kg/m^2$. The precise mechanism for this association is not fully understood, although it is increasingly recognized that the sequence of obesity leading to sleep apnea, which is a strong risk factor for atrial fibrillation and thereby stroke, may account for some of the observed risk.

Alongside the independent risk, obesity increases stroke risk through its association with many classical vascular risk factors (hypertension, left ventricular hypertrophy, diabetes, and dyslipidemia), which may usefully be addressed on their own merits in tandem with interventions to promote weight loss. Good control of cardiovascular risk factors, including anticoagulation where appropriate for atrial fibrillation, is a key intervention for the prevention of stroke.

Obesity and CHF

Epidemiological studies into the relationship between obesity and heart failure are hampered by the fact that many patients with significant heart failure become cachectic, thereby obscuring the causal relationship. Furthermore, there is a paradox in the prognosis in heart failure. Once CHF is established, the prognosis tends to be better in those with higher rather than lower BMI. Studies need to be careful to avoid labeling individuals with peripheral edema as having heart failure without considering the other causes of this common physical sign in obesity. Notwithstanding these difficulties, it is thought that for each BMI unit over $25\,kg/m^2$, the risk of heart failure increases by some 5–7% with overweight being associated with 20–50% increased risk and obesity with an approximate doubling of heart failure risk.

It is thought that cardiac failure in obesity derives from remodeling of the heart in response to pressure and volume stresses, particularly in a context of atherogenic risk factors for coronary artery disease and over-activation of the SNS. This is particularly evident where obesity is complicated by OSA. The outcome is a mixture of eccentric hypertrophy followed by dilation and eventually failure, which is pathologically distinct from that seen in pure pressure (e.g., hypertension) or volume (e.g., valvular incompetence) induced remodeling. This particular pattern has been termed "obesity cardiomyopathy."

The presence of left ventricular hypertrophy is an adverse prognostic indicator, better than either systolic or diastolic blood pressure for predicting mortality. However, there is good evidence that weight loss of the order of 8 kg in obese individuals can reduce blood pressure by 13/14 mmHg and reduce left ventricular mass by as much as 20% and exercise may yield additional benefit.

Obesity and sudden death

Obesity increases the risk of sudden death. A variety of mechanisms have been suggested, which include increased SNS activity, prolongation of the QT interval, and structural heart disease such as coronary artery disease and obesity-related cardiomyopathy. The risk of sudden death is increased by the presence of risk factors for coronary heart disease (by a factor of

2.5–4.0-fold for smoking, hypertension, and diabetes) and is also increased independently by a factor of around 1.6 by being obese. Most of these sudden deaths are thought to be due to arrhythmias, and it seems likely that individuals with an inherited susceptibility (e.g., ion channelopathy) are particularly vulnerable to the effects of QTc prolongation by, for example, diuretics, laxatives, other medications, very-low-calorie diets that have been associated with sudden death in some but not all studies, or activation of the SNS (as in OSA). There is preliminary evidence that, apart from avoiding aggravating factors in susceptible individuals, consumption of long- and intermediate-chain essential polyunsaturated fatty acids may confer some degree of protection against sudden cardiac death in obesity.

Management of cardiovascular risk in obesity

Presentation of coronary heart disease in obesity is highly variable, ranging from asymptomatic undiagnosed disease to sudden cardiac death. Whereas the development of a first vascular event identifies a group of patients with a markedly increased risk of further adverse outcomes, one of the greatest difficulties facing the clinician is in recognizing the much larger number of individuals with clinically silent disease and intervening appropriately to prevent first events.

Patients with obesity should be screened for cardiovascular risk factors on a regular basis by their primary care practitioners. These risk factors include hypertension, diabetes, impaired fasting glucose or impaired glucose tolerance, and hyperlipidemia. It is increasingly recognized that ED in the metabolic syndrome may be an early warning of a more global atherosclerotic vascular disease. Advice should be given where appropriate on smoking cessation and support and advice offered to promote weight loss. Although weight loss may be beneficial for several obesity-related risk factors, effective pharmacologic interventions should not be delayed pending failure of unrealistic weight loss ambitions. Weight loss if maintained long term appears to be associated with increased life span (Figure 17.2).

Aerobic exercise of moderate intensity can reduce the CVD risk independent of any associated weight loss, and lack of weight loss should not put off individuals with obesity from carrying out regular exercise.

OSA should be actively considered in all obese individuals, especially where there is refractory hypertension or daytime somnolence. The prevalence of this condition may approach or even exceed 50% in class III obesity.

Low-dose aspirin is currently mainly recommended for those with a previous cardiovascular event rather than in primary prevention strategies

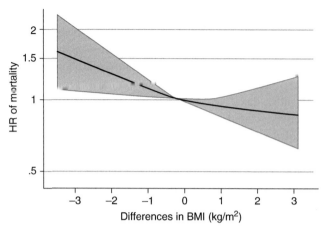

Figure 17.2 HRs and 95% confidence intervals of mortality according to differences in body mass index (DBMI) with adjustment for differences in waist circumference (DWC). Reproduced from Berentzen *et al.* [1], with permission from the Public Library of Science.

for vascular disease. The use of cardiovascular risk calculators (many, including the Framingham or UKPDS risk calculators, are available online) enables estimation of approximate 10-year cardiovascular event risks taking into account an individual's known cardiovascular risk factors. Such risk calculators enable rational decisions to be made around the use of, for example, statin therapy in primary prevention where the potential risk–benefit ratio depends on the patient's individual risk of suffering a vascular event within a specific time frame.

Where obesity is complicated by hypertension, weight loss is associated with an improvement in blood pressure. The management of hypertension in this situation should always start with lifestyle advice centered on diet and exercise along with salt and alcohol restriction. Management then needs to be individualized depending on overall risk and clinical and demographic circumstances. Examples include the use of diuretics and calcium antagonists in the elderly or Afro-Caribbean patients and the use of beta-blockers and calcium antagonists in those with ischemic heart disease. Most patients will require combination anti-hypertension drug therapy. Obese patients with T2DM or impaired glucose tolerance have a reduced risk of cardiovascular events when prescribed metformin, which is seen independent of the weight loss that this drug causes.

With its increasing availability and safety and in the context of evidence that bariatric surgery results in significant weight loss sustained over the long term, this is an option that should be considered by some individuals with higher BMI and increased cardiovascular risk, particularly in the context of T2DM or failure of conventional treatments.

Pitfalls

1. Over-estimating blood pressure using an inappropriately narrow cuff.

2. Obesity is often also associated with NAFLD and abnormal LFTs. Statins are not contra-indicated in these patients, and with weight loss and better control of lipids, LFTs often improve.

3. Delaying effective treatments for cardiovascular risk factors pending non-achievement of unrealistic weight loss goals. In many cases, therapy may more effectively be withdrawn after the patient achieves weight loss goals rather than be withheld unreasonably at the outset.

4. Failure to consider the effects of drugs and electrolyte abnormalities that may lengthen QTc, especially in high-risk patients.

5. Not considering a diagnosis of OSA in patients with obesity. It is very common (perhaps 50% prevalence in class III obesity) and a major contributor to resistant hypertension and cardiovascular risk.

Key web links

Framingham Heart Study Risk Score. http://www.framinghamheartstudy.org/risk/index.html [accessed on December 29, 2012].

United Kingdom Prospective Diabetes Study (UKPDS). *Risk Engine*. http://www.dtu.ox.ac.uk/riskengine/ [accessed on December 29, 2012].

Reference

1 Berentzen, T.L., Jakobsen, M.U., Halkjaer, J., Tjønneland, A., Overvad, K. & Sørensen, T.I. (2010) Changes in waist circumference and mortality in middle-aged men and women. *PLoS One.* 5, e13097.

Further reading

Adler, A.I., Stratton, I.M., Neil, H.A.W. *et al.* (2000) Association of systolic blood pressure with macrovascular and microvascular complications of type 2 diabetes (UKPDS 36): Prospective observational study. *BMJ*, 321, 412.

Berrington de Gonzalez, A., Hartge, P., Cerhan, J.R. *et al.* (2010) Body-mass index and mortality among 1.46 million white adults. *New England Journal of Medicine*, 363, 2211–2219.

Kenchaiah, S., Evans, J.C., Levy, D. *et al.* (2002) Obesity and the risk of heart failure. *New England Journal of Medicine*, 347, 305–313.

Modan, M., Almog, S., Fuchs, Z., Chetrit, A., Lusky, A. & Halkin, H. (1991) Obesity, glucose intolerance, hyperinsulinemia and response to anti-hypertensive drugs. *Hypertension*, 17, 565–573.

Palatini, P., Saladini, F., Mos, L. *et al.* (2012) Obesity is a strong determinant of hypertensive target organ damage in young-to-middle-age patients. *International Journal of Obesity (London)*, doi: 10.1038/ijo.2012.32.

Prospective Studies Collaboration. (2009) Body-mass index and cause-specific mortality in 900,000 adults: Collaborative analysis of 57 prospective studies. *Lancet,* 373, 1083–1096.

Schottede, D.E. & Stunkard, A.J. (1990) The effects of weight reduction on blood pressure in 301 obese patients. *Archives of Internal Medicine,* 150, 1701–1704.

Sullivan, M., Karlsson, J., Sjöström, L. *et al.* (1993) Swedish obese subjects (SOS) – an intervention study of obesity. Baseline evaluation of health and psychosocial functioning in the first 1743 subjects examined. *International Journal of Obesity and Related Metabolic Disorders,* 17, 503–512.

CHAPTER 18

Obesity: Mental Health and Social Consequences

Key points

- There is systematic and widespread stigma associated with obesity including discrimination, stereotyping, and unequal treatment in society today. Consequently, low self-esteem, increased anxiety, and depression are widespread in patients with obesity.
- Obese individuals are usually labeled "lazy" and lacking self-control. In health-care settings, obese patients often face discrimination when they require health interventions.
- Obesity is more prevalent in lower socio-economic groups. Obese individuals are disadvantaged in virtually all aspects of social activity, including education, employment, health care, and interpersonal relationships.
- It is important to consider psychological and emotional support for obese patients. Their health beliefs influence how they may respond to different options for lifestyle modification. The clinician must explore the patient's mental well-being and also identify social factors that may be causing the patient distress.
- There is a high rate of use of prescription medication for anxiety and depression in Western societies, and many of these promote weight gain.

CASE STUDIES

Case study 1

DM, a 22-year-old college student, was bullied since childhood for being overweight. She lacked self-esteem and confidence. When her roommate moved out with her boyfriend, she became depressed and agoraphobic and gained 20 lb in 4 weeks.

Comment: She was referred to a cognitive behavior therapist. After six sessions of therapy, she learned techniques to cope with her situation and her feelings. She then engaged more in active weight management and lost 20 lb in 2 months. She is now more confident about herself and has more self-esteem, and she continues to lose weight.

Practical Manual of Clinical Obesity, First Edition. Robert Kushner, Victor Lawrence and Sudhesh Kumar.
© 2013 John Wiley & Sons, Ltd. Published 2013 by John Wiley & Sons, Ltd.

> **Case study 2**
>
> *LP, a 42-year-old unemployed woman, attended the obesity clinic. She has been obese since the age of 13 and currently weighs 240 lb with a BMI of 41 kg/m². She does not have diabetes or hypertension but suffers from anxiety and depression and has failed numerous attempts at losing weight.*
>
> **Comment**: Further questioning revealed that she had been sexually abused during her early teenage years by her mother's boyfriend. She visited a psychologist who explored these issues with her and helped her understand that she had been sub-consciously trying to look unattractive since she was a teenager. She is now dealing with these issues and was then able to lose 15 lb over the following 4 months.

Principles for management

Obesity and culture

The social environment is a major determinant of obesity allowing the realization of one's genetic potential. Environment includes the social and cultural context in which people live. A large study of the role of social networks from the Framingham Heart Study in influencing obesity in individuals suggested a person's social network is more closely linked to their BMI than their family members whom they are not socially close to. Also of interest is the way society and culture can influence the perception of body weight in different cultures. Obesity is considered a disease and is socially stigmatized in Western society, yet in some other cultures, "big is beautiful." Indeed, in these societies, being lean may be considered a sign of occult disease or poor social status. These social attitudes may affect an individual's mental well-being.

There is a significant effect of socio-economic status on the prevalence of obesity. As a generalization, obesity afflicts "poor people in rich countries and rich people in poor countries." This is particularly the case in low- and middle-income countries in transition to a Western society. Here, there is a double burden of infectious diseases and of chronic diseases associated with obesity. Initially, these changes are seen with urbanization and resultant reduced physical activity and increased consumption of an energy-dense diet.

An important implication of culture and the social context of obesity is first to encourage professionals and patients and their families to avoid medicalizing large sections of their adult population and instead consider the effect on co-morbid diseases, such as diabetes and heart disease. Further, clinicians must be mindful of the cultural and social context of the patients in order to better understand how to manage obesity and related disorders in these individuals.

The stigma associated with obesity and implications for management

The popular belief among the general public, reflected also among politicians and policy makers, is that obesity is self-inflicted and can be reversed by personally controlled behavior alone. The fact that obesity is the result of a complex interplay of factors and that biology and the environment have major roles in its causation is often not clear even to the obese individual. To make matters worse, there are often repeated episodes of weight loss followed by regain of weight that is seen as a failure on the part of the individual. Therefore, professionals managing obesity should be wary that while it is important to provide information about controllable aspects of obesity, it may have an unintended consequence in emphasizing the negative stereotype of weight control. Many patients find it helpful to put this in the context of underlying biological tendencies and environmental factors, like their job, for example.

Obesity and mental illness

Addressing the low self-esteem and stigma related to obesity is clearly important to achieve the best overall goals for obese children and adults. Unfortunately, this requires the understanding and participation of a very wide range of people from home to work. Thus, obesity can be a challenge for the individual to live with every day, as unlike many other medical conditions that can be kept personal, the obese state is obvious to anyone. Therefore, despite good work from health professionals or family, it is often impossible to avoid such individuals facing obstacles that can impair their QOL due to the bias they may face. Support from family and friends and professionals can assist obese patients in managing their emotional state and to help them continue to participate positively in all aspects of life in society. The management of obesity in the current obesity epidemic has sociocultural implications. Four paradigms for the management are summarized in Table 18.1. Support from the health professional along with family and friends is required to overcome the stigma of obesity to improve the chances of weight loss.

Obesity is associated with higher rates of anxiety and depression. Anxiety disorders are 1.5–1.68 times more prevalent in patients with obesity compared to lean patients. Mood disorders are about 1.25–1.6 times more common in patients with obesity. In many cases, this may require treatment in its own right and may not simply be expected to resolve itself during weight management. In the Hoorn Diabetes Study, the number of major stressful life events during a preceding 5-year period was associated with rates of abdominal obesity and a higher risk of undiagnosed diabetes.

Table 18.1 The four paradigms of obesity.

Paradigm characteristics	Moral	Medical	Sociopolitical	Globopolitical
Paradigm reach	Wide	Medium	Small and select	Global
Perception of body fat	Bad, sinful, ugly	Promotes illness	A fact	Present in epidemic proportions
Perception of a fat person	Weak Lacks willpower	Have an illness beyond their control	Member of society	Disdain Discrimination
Relationship with society	Burden on society	Society a source of harm (e.g., excess calories)	Confrontational	Affliction of the century
Responsibility for fat condition	Personal blame	An illness Neutral but not value free	None	Maladaptation All are at risk
Language	Fat, corpulent, plump	Obese, adipose, overweight	Large, ample, of size	Fat, socially/sexually unattractive (female) Slob, "fat bastard" (male)
Eating	Gluttony, gorging	Acoria, polyphagia, hyperorexia	A pleasurable social activity	Vigilance required All are at risk
Activity	Sloth, laziness	Lethargy, listlessness	Neutral	Sedentary

Reaction to a fat person	Stigmatization Discrimination Disdain	Stigma of sickness and disability Dependent on medical expertise	Accept large people as normal	Mortality risk Drain on health budget
Legitimizing experts	Religious or traditional	Scientific or clinical	Selected scientists and social scientists	Medical and other clinical obesity specialists
Organizations/industries supporting paradigm	Fashion, cosmetic Weight loss	Health care Pharmaceutical Weight loss	Selected magazines, books	Medical and other clinical obesity specialists
	Sport, activity	Sport, activity	Specialized fashions	Pharmaceutical Weight loss Fashion, cosmetic Media
Solution focus	Fat person's willpower and determination	Treatment with medical supervision	Change society's attitudes	Preventive focus, especially for children
			Fat liberation	Realistic expectations

A number of studies have shown chronic stress as an independent risk factor for obesity. Depression and anxiety are also risk factors for poorer prognosis in weight management programs. Often this is also linked to poor socio-economic circumstances, making the management of these patients rather difficult. Thus, these patients may require cognitive behavior therapy for this before embarking on treatment with drugs or surgery. However, often losing weight successfully (including with bariatric surgery) is associated with improvement in symptoms of depression and anxiety. Thus, there is a complex bi-directional relationship between obesity and psychological functioning, and a skilled professional psychologist is often required in order to untie the Gordian knot.

There is a U-shaped relationship between obesity and Alzheimer's disease that has now been borne out in a number of studies. The studies of longer duration show the strongest association with obesity with an increased risk of about 42% compared to normal-weight individuals.

Obesity and major psychiatric diseases

Obesity in an individual with major psychiatric illness, such as schizophrenia or psychosis, can be extremely difficult to manage. The prognosis depends on the degree of control of the underlying psychiatric illness. The management of these patients becomes even more challenging because the majority of drugs used to manage these conditions result in aggravation of obesity, for example, tricyclic anti-depressants, lithium, olanzapine, and risperidone. Development of newer anti-psychotic agents that are less likely to cause obesity is an ongoing field of research. In these patients, the carers need to be educated on regulating the environment so there is less access to calorie-dense food and opportunities for healthy diet and exercise are available to the patient. Nevertheless, in these cases, mitigating weight gain is sometimes the best that one can offer.

Obesity and mental well-being in children

The impact of obesity-related stigma can be severe for obese children, having deleterious emotional and physical health consequences. There is evidence that weight-based teasing is associated with poorer psychological outcomes among both male and female adolescents. What is more worrying is that obesity-related teasing and bullying is associated with increased risk for suicide. Several large population-based studies have demonstrated that obese adolescents are more likely than non-obese to consider or attempt suicide. Obesity also appears to affect academic performance and achievement adversely.

One consequence of teasing and bullying at school is eating disorders. Thus, behaviors such as binge eating, vomiting, bulimia, and the use of diet pills or laxatives do not develop in a vacuum, they are associated with being teased or bullied because of overweight/obesity. There is a need for more research to see if successful intervention programs to reduce stigmatization of overweight in childhood might reduce psychological morbidity that could last lifelong.

Management

Mental well-being and social difficulties should be explored during consultation by at least one member of the clinical team. A number of tools can be used to screen patients for anxiety or depression prior to a consultation. Questionnaire-based tools such as the Hospital Anxiety and Depression Scale (HADS) are often used and those with a high HADS score are then assessed in more detail. A history of very distressing life events, going back to childhood, can point to significant underlying psychological issues that may need to be dealt with before successful weight management can be achieved in many cases.

Use of anti-depressants is very common among patients with obesity. Unfortunately, most of these promote weight gain and should only be used where there is no non-pharmacologic alternative. Chapter 10 describes some techniques that could be helpful here, and positive results with weight management can help improve the patients' mood and anxiety levels.

Pitfalls

- Abuse during childhood can be quite common in adults presenting with obesity, and such individuals may require psychological intervention. This may sometimes be overlooked but needs to be dealt with for the successful management of obesity.
- In obese individuals of ethnic minority backgrounds, it is important to understand cultural differences that may affect the clinical management.
- Use of anti-depressants is often associated with weight gain, which could further aggravate the problem.
- The patient's occupation and the behavior of others in the workplace can affect success of weight management programs. Sometimes individuals with obesity are moved from an active job to one where they sit behind a desk for concern around health and safety. However, this change may make things worse.

Key web link

National Obesity Observatory UK, Obesity and Mental Health Briefing Paper. http://www.noo.org.uk/NOO_pub/briefing_papers [accessed on December 29 2012].

Further reading

Atlantis, E., Goldney, R.D. & Wittert, G.A. (2009) Obesity and depression or anxiety. *BMJ*, 339, b3868.

Brown, P.J. (1992) The biocultural evolution of obesity: an anthropological view. In: P. Bjorntorp & B. N. Brodoff (eds), *Obesity*, pp. 320–329. JB Lippincott, Philadelphia.

Chandola, T., Brunner, E. & Marmot, M. (2006) Chronic stress at work and the metabolic syndrome: Prospective study. *BMJ*, 332, 521–525.

Christakis, N.A. & Fowler, J.H. (2007) The spread of obesity in a large social network over 32 years. *New England Journal of Medicine*, 357, 370–379.

Kivimäki, M., Lawlor, D.A., Singh-Manoux, A. *et al.* (2009) Common mental disorder and obesity: Insight from four repeat measures over 19 years: Prospective Whitehall II cohort study. *BMJ*, 339, b3765.

Legenbauer, T., De Zwaan, M., Benecke, A., Muhlhans, B., Petrak, F. & Herpertz, S. (2009) Depression and anxiety: Their predictive function for weight loss in obese individuals. *Obesity Facts*, 2, 227–234.

Profenno, L.A., Porsteinsson, A.P. & Faraone, S.V. (2010) Meta-analysis of Alzheimer's disease risk with obesity, diabetes, and related disorders. *Biological Psychiatry*, 67, 505–512.

Williams, N. (2008) *Managing Obesity in the Workplace*. Radcliffe Publishing, Oxford.

Zigmond, A.S. & Snaith, R.P. (1983) The hospital anxiety and depression scale. *Acta Psychiatrica Scandinavia*, 67, 361–370.

CHAPTER 19

Obesity and Musculo-skeletal Disease

Key points

- Obesity is associated with an increased risk of musculo-skeletal disorders including osteoarthritis and gout.
- Obesity *per se* can increase disability, primarily due to osteoarthritis. Obesity is associated with gout especially when other metabolic disorders (such as metabolic syndrome) are also present. A combination of obesity and widespread osteoarthritis can be a challenge for the patient to live with and for the clinician to treat.
- Obese patients should not be excluded from having knee or hip replacement simply because of obesity. However, outcomes for these people are not as good as for individuals without obesity, and people with obesity are at higher risk of deep vein venous thrombosis and pulmonary embolism following surgery.
- Preventing musculo-skeletal disorders through anticipatory action is better than trying to treat it in people with obesity.

CASE STUDIES

Case study 1

JM is a 45-year-old man with rheumatoid arthritis diagnosed at the age of 25. He has been on courses of steroids multiple times over the past years. His mobility has progressively worsened over the last 10 years, and he now needs a walking stick to leave the house. His weight has also been progressively increasing over the years and he now weighs 360 lb, giving him a BMI of 55 kg/m². He has now also been diagnosed to have osteoarthritis of hips and knees.

Comment: Recent scans confirm degenerative changes in his spine, which cause severe back pain. He has failed in several previous attempts at weight loss, but more recently with the help of a weight management counselor, he undertook a very-low-calorie diet of 800 kcal/day. He lost 30 lb in 3 months and this has relieved some of the pain, especially in his back. He can now go for short walks in the backyard. He continues to lose weight, although not as rapidly as when he first started his diet, and he is now

---

Practical Manual of Clinical Obesity, First Edition. Robert Kushner, Victor Lawrence and Sudhesh Kumar.
© 2013 John Wiley & Sons, Ltd. Published 2013 by John Wiley & Sons, Ltd.

on a low-calorie diet. He manages to walk for a few minutes several times each day and feels confident that he can continue his current diet and activity regime. However, he still suffers from severe pains in his hands and knee joints that he has secondary to his arthritis.

Case study 2

PL is a 55-year-old lady with long-standing obesity, and she has had progressively worsening joint pains, predominantly in her right hip and left knee. She has seen an orthopedic surgeon who recommended a right hip replacement but declined to operate before she lost weight. She weighed 280 lb that made her BMI 48 kg/m², and she also had a past history of deep vein thrombosis.

Comment: She started a weight management program, and she subsequently had a sleeve gastrectomy following which she lost over 50 lb. She then successfully underwent a hip replacement and is able to walk better allowing her to do more exercise. She is doing well and continues to lose weight, although she still suffers from pain in her other joints.

Obesity and musculo-skeletal disease

With the increasing worldwide prevalence of obesity, there is also an increasing worldwide burden of musculo-skeletal problems, especially in the Western world. The increase in obesity has been linked to the rapid rise in osteoarthritis mainly of weight-bearing joints including the knee, hip, ankle, and foot. Obesity is also related to the rise in conditions such as gout, rheumatoid arthritis, spondyloarthropathy, back pain, and fibromyalgia. Vitamin D deficiency has also been shown to be more common in obesity. The increase in mortality with obesity related to CVD, cancers, respiratory disease, and diabetes has taken most of the attention of public health policies with relatively less importance given to the rise in musculoskeletal disorders related to obesity. However, although there is a limited impact on mortality, there is a huge morbidity and cost implication of obesity and musculo-skeletal disorders. There is an increase in the direct cost due to a greater need for joint replacement surgery. However, the much bigger indirect cost is of pain related to musculo-skeletal problems, leading to days off work, reduced productivity, and lower QOL. In Europe, musculo-skeletal pain has been classed as the most expensive of all disease categories. It is second to only CVDs in the USA and Australia, although indirect costs are thought to be much higher. Although there is a lot of focus on osteoarthritis and joint problems related to obesity, bones and soft tissue, including tendons, cartilage, and menisci, are also affected by obesity. There is also an effect of obesity in childhood and adolescence on the growing skeleton, both structurally and functionally, although there is a paucity of long-term data. Paradoxically, there seems to be a reduced risk of hip and wrist fracture in elderly individuals with obesity. This may be due to increased regional bone mineral density in obese individuals as well as a greater cushioning effect of the surrounding fat pad. There may be an effect of reduced mobility in individuals with obesity, which further contributes to this reduced fracture risk.

Obesity and osteoarthritis

Osteoarthritis is more common in patients with obesity. The risk for osteoarthritis of the knee is almost fourfold in obese women and 4.8-fold in obese men compared to people with a normal BMI, based on data from the first National Health and Nutrition Examination Survey I (NHANES I). This may partly be because of the increased mechanical load and abnormal stresses on the joints. However, degenerative arthritis in obesity is not merely a consequence of mechanical stress due to excess weight. There is now ample evidence that systemic factors related to the obese state may also play a role, especially adipocytokines and chronic inflammation (Figure 19.1). For example, the hormone leptin that is elevated in human obesity is linked to direct damage to chondrocytes. Other hypotheses include deficiencies in diet, including high fat content that may damage the bone and cartilage. Vitamin D deficiency is also more common in the obese. These observations may also help explain higher rates of arthritis of small joints in the hands in addition to the weight-bearing joints in obesity. Arthritis in an obese individual may progress more rapidly because of the downward spiral of inactivity and further joint damage. Most of the disability associated with obesity is probably related to the presence of co-morbidities including diabetes, vascular disease, or sleep apnea, but obesity *per se* is also associated with increased disability. The presence of lymphedema aggravates the difficulty with mobility further.

Obesity and gout

Serum uric acid levels are elevated in the obese, particularly where other features of metabolic syndrome are present. The prevalence of gout as well as hyperuricemia in the USA according to NHANES 2007–2008 showed a significant increase with 3.9% of the population diagnosed to have gout (8.3 million people) and an age-adjusted rise of 1.0% compared to NHANES 1988–1994. Adjustment for BMI greatly reduced this increase, suggesting an increase in obesity as a reason for this increase in cases of gout as well as of hyperuricemia.

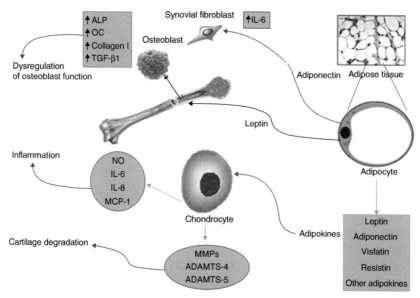

Figure 19.1 Schematic representation of the complex network that links WAT dysfunction, bone, and cartilage tissues. Dysfunctional fat produces an excess of pro-inflammatory adipokines that are able to interact with bone cells, synovial cells, and chondrocytes by inducing pro-inflammatory mediators (cytokines, ROS, NO) and cartilage degradation factors (metalloproteases and ADAMTSs). Reproduced from Conde *et al. Arthritis* 2011; 2011:203901.

Obesity and low back pain

Low back pain is common in individuals with obesity. A recent meta-analysis has shown an increased risk in individuals with obesity compared to those with a normal BMI of having low back pain in the last 12 months (odds ratio 1.33), seeking care for low back pain (odds ratio 1.56), and having chronic low back pain (odds ratio 1.53). The benefit of various exercise programs or physical activity to improve symptoms is debatable, possibly partly due to the associated weight loss in some studies and not in others. Significant weight loss, if achieved, does result in reduction in low back pain, and there is evidence from several studies of an improvement in low back pain following weight loss with bariatric surgery.

Management algorithms

Weight loss does result in improvement of symptoms, especially pain, in most musculo-skeletal conditions in individuals with obesity. This should be the aim of management in these individuals. However, weight loss *per se* has not been shown to cure existing arthritis. There is some evidence of a reduction in reported pain in knee osteoarthritis following significant weight reduction with bariatric surgery from 54% to 14% following weight loss of 100 lb. There is stronger evidence, however, of change in risk of developing new osteoarthritis with change in BMI. The Framingham Heart Study showed that a decrease in BMI of 2 kg/m^2 or more over a period of 10 years could reduce the odds of developing new osteoarthritis of the knee by over 50%. Conversely, weight gain is associated with a higher risk of osteoarthritis. It has been estimated that the risk of knee osteoarthritis increases by 35% for every 11 lb of weight gained. Therefore, prevention of new osteoarthritis can be achieved by weight management strategies early on.

Referral to relevant professionals such as physiotherapists and occupational therapists can be very helpful to the patient with arthritis restricting mobility. Analgesia is the mainstay of treatment, and good pain management with referral for exercise programs is the best option. Unfortunately, most people with arthritis are fearful of physical activity due to the pain and fear of worsening the joints. There is usually an increasing need for stronger analgesics with time and reducing mobility, leading to a downward spiral of reducing mobility and increasing obesity, often associated with depression and a low QOL. Use of appropriate aids can help with mobility and greater independence. Activities like swimming can be easier for patients with arthritis where buoyancy in water allows more movement without the joints having to bear the full weight of the body.

Joint replacement surgery is often not offered to patients with obesity, partly because outcomes are not as good as for individuals without obesity and partly because of the higher anesthetic risk and risk of deep vein thrombosis or pulmonary embolism post-operatively. However, a risk–benefit analysis must be done and surgery should not be denied to all patients with obesity. Some patients undergo very-low-calorie or low-calorie diet regimens or even bariatric surgery to lose weight in preparation for joint replacement surgery, leading to better outcomes.

In rheumatoid arthritis, newer therapies may cause less weight gain than corticosteroid therapy. Vitamin D deficiency is easily treated with vitamin D replacement with calcium supplements. When gout is diagnosed, fundamental changes to diet and alcohol should be advised together with reduction in ingestion of purine-rich foods, like beef, liver, and soya beans. Allopurinol should be prescribed to prevent acute gout attacks, and treatment of hypertension as well as weight loss strategies must be undertaken concurrently.

Pitfalls

- Obesity management must commence early as soon as evidence of arthritis is seen in an overweight individual. Prevention is much easier than treatment. Neither the patient nor the clinician must ignore signs of arthritis early on.
- Vitamin D levels must be checked in all patients with obesity and any deficiency corrected.
- Increase in activity and exercise should always be encouraged with the use of analgesia where necessary to avoid a downward spiral due to ever-increasing difficulties with mobility and a sense of hopelessness.
- Taking up swimming or making small changes such as standing more often than sitting can contribute to weight loss. Small changes can help, and often patients feel the need to try more drastic physical exercise, which may risk damage to joints and reduce mobility.
- With the use of NSAIDs for pain relief to relieve pain in arthritis, patients should be made aware and monitored for signs or symptoms of upper GI bleeds and ulcers as well as renal impairment. Anti-depressants can also be useful in those with chronic pain.

Key web link

http://www.hopkinsarthritis.org/patient-corner/disease-management/role-of-body-weight-in-osteoarthritis/ [accessed on December 29, 2012].

Further reading

Blagojevic, M., Jinks, C., Jeffery, A. & Jordan, K.P. (2010) Risk factors for onset of osteoarthritis of the knee in older adults: A systematic review and meta-analysis. *Osteoarthritis Cartilage*, 18, 24–33.

Gelber, A.C., Hochberg, M.C., Mead, L.A., Wang, N.Y., Wigley, F.M. & Klag, M.J. (1999) Body mass index in young men and the risk of subsequent knee and hip osteoarthritis. *American Journal of Medicine*, 107, 542–548.

Hart, H.D. & Spector, T.D. (1993) The relationship between obesity, fat distribution and osteoarthritis in women in the general population with 10 years follow up. *Journal of Rheumatology*, 20, 331–335.

Kyrou, I., Osei-Assibey, G., Williams, N. *et al.* (2011) Self-reported disability in adults with severe obesity. *Journal of Obesity*, 2011, 918402.

Lievense, A.M., Bierma-Zeinstra, S.M., Verhagen, A.P., van Baar, M.E., Verhaar, J.A. & Koes, B.W. (2002) Influence of obesity on the development of osteoarthritis of the hip: A systematic review. *Rheumatology (Oxford)*, 41, 1155–1162.

Shiri, R., Karppinen, J., Leino-Arjas, P., Solovieva, S. & Viikari-Juntura, E. (2010) The association between obesity and low back pain: A meta-analysis. *American Journal of Epidemiology*, 171(2), 135–154.

Wearing, S.C., Hennig, E.M., Byrne, N.M., Steele, J.R. & Hills, A.P. (2006) Musculoskeletal disorders associated with obesity: A biomechanical perspective. *Obesity Reviews*, 7, 239–250.

Zhu, Y., Pandya, B.J. & Choi, H.K. (2011) Prevalence of gout and hyperuricemia in the US general population: The National Health and Nutrition Examination Survey 2007–2008. *Arthritis & Rheumatism*, 63, 3136–3141.

CHAPTER 20

The Obese Patient in Hospital

Key points

- Due to the high prevalence of obesity in society, it is fairly common to have patients with morbid obesity and other medical problems admitted in hospital.
- Hospitals must therefore invest in appropriate infrastructure to cater for patients with extreme obesity in waiting rooms, hospital wards, theaters, emergency departments, and ambulances.
- Taking good care of a patient with extreme obesity as an inpatient requires changes to virtually all services offered in the hospital. Early identification of such patients with extreme obesity is essential.

CASE STUDIES

Case study 1

SD, a 30-year-old lady with a weight of 350 lb and a BMI of 60 kg/m², attended the antenatal clinic during her second trimester. None of the chairs in the waiting room were wide enough for her to sit in, and she had to sit across two chairs. Her weight could not be recorded as the scale did not go above 300 lb.

Comment: She had an elective admission at 41 weeks for a planned induction of labor and was surprised that the nursing staff had to borrow an appropriate bed for her from another ward. She had a normal vaginal delivery, but made a formal complaint to the hospital following her discharge about how the hospital was not prepared for her admission and treatment.

Case study 2

RP, a 35-year-old man with a weight of 450 lb and a BMI of 71 kg/m2, was admitted to hospital with central chest pain. There was a delay in his arrival to the emergency department because of the difficulty of moving him from his house to the ambulance. It took six staff members to move him on to a bed in the department, and he was upset when he overheard one of the staff commenting to a colleague that she had probably hurt her back when moving him. It took the doctor six attempts to obtain intravenous access, and his chest pain had subsided by this time. There was another long delay in

---

Practical Manual of Clinical Obesity, First Edition. Robert Kushner, Victor Lawrence and Sudhesh Kumar.
© 2013 John Wiley & Sons, Ltd. Published 2013 by John Wiley & Sons, Ltd.

transferring him to a ward for overnight observation, because of lack of a suitable wheelchair and an appropriate bed in the ward. He had a normal ECG and normal troponin I, and he was discharged the next day following overnight observation.

Comment: He gave an interview to the local newspaper the following week about his poor care in hospital, although the medical management of his chest pain had been faultless.

The obese patient in hospital

There is an increasing prevalence of obesity worldwide, and the prevalence of morbid obesity (BMI > 40 kg/m^2) is also increasing. The American Society for Metabolic and Bariatric Surgery estimates that 220,000 patients underwent bariatric surgery in 2009 in the USA alone. There is a high likelihood of any hospital having an inpatient that weighs more than 300 lb at any given time. Although some patients may be admitted for bariatric surgery in special wards and have dedicated theater tables, patients with morbid obesity are also likely to be admitted for emergency surgery for other illnesses and the need for specialist facilities becomes apparent. They may also be admitted to general wards and departments for other acute medical problems, and similarly, the issue of facilities and specialist support for their obesity is raised as a matter of urgency. Many patients with morbid obesity also attend the outpatient departments, and usual facilities for patients such as chairs, weighing scales, and even doors are not fit for the purpose.

Specialist equipment for the morbidly obese

As inpatients, every service in the hospital will encounter patients with morbid obesity, and standard chairs, beds, gowns, or theater tables are not adequate. A lot of CT and MRI scanners have a maximum internal diameter, meaning severely obese patients do not fit in these. The tables on the scanners also have a maximum weight, as do operating theater tables and regular hospital beds. Even structures like doors may not be wide enough for the patient or their wide bed/wheelchair. A full list of appliances and services affected is listed in Table 20.1. When patients are too heavy or big for standard appliances, it causes embarrassment to the patients and frustration to the treating staff. Injury to the patient or staff could result if staff try to lift or move these patients in the absence of suitable equipment. This could result in days lost from work and long-term sickness among staff as well as the possible cost of litigation if the patient is injured.

Table 20.1 List of services or appliances that need modification for the appropriate management of patients with severe obesity.

Special weighing scales including chairs and beds that can weigh heavier patients

Extra-wide gowns

Wider chairs preferably without arms

Appropriate hoists and lifts

Wider wheelchairs that sustain the extra weight

Beds that are wider and sustain the extra weight

Appropriate pressure relief mattresses

Appropriate toilets and bathrooms with extra space

CT and MRI scanners that have an open top or larger internal diameter and that can take the extra weight

Wider theater tables that sustain the extra weight

Wider doors to accommodate the wider beds and chairs

Wider ramps for wheelchairs and beds

Ambulances with wider doors and appropriate trolleys

Appliances that are suitable for the extremely obese patient are very expensive, and estimates are that the USA may have spent $1.2 billion by the end of 2011 purchasing these supplies. It is not feasible to have all hospital beds and chairs suitable for the severely obese patients, and this is where pre-planning and awareness of managers are important. The minimum numbers of appliances required for a hospital or clinical practice must be identified, and they must be stored in a pre-planned ward or space so that they can be accessed when necessary. Outpatient departments should have some chairs that are suitable for those with severe obesity, as well as armless chairs. Patients undergoing elective surgery attend pre-operative anesthetic checks, and those needing special equipment should be identified so that the staff are prepared when the patient arrives in the department. Departments involved in the care of patients that undergo bariatric surgery are more likely to have suitable equipment, and staff from these wards can help by lending equipment or giving training and advice. All hospital staff should be trained on how to use this equipment as well as on health and safety regulations to avoid injuring themselves. Wide gowns, wider wheelchairs, wider examination couches, wider beds and trolleys, and special scales are some of the equipment that would be needed in most wards on a regular basis. All hospitals should have a nominated person responsible for training staff, carrying out risk assessments as well as ensuring the right equipment is available or can be borrowed from a previously identified area or supplier.

Emergency care

Planning for elective admissions and surgical procedures is possible but not for attendances in the emergency department. All emergency departments should have plans of how to deal with a severely obese patient that attends the department. A study in Ireland showed that none of the emergency departments questioned had adequate infrastructure or equipment to deal with the admission of a severely obese patient.

Patients with severe obesity are more likely to suffer from medical complications, as discussed in other chapters in this book. Subsequently, these individuals are more likely to be admitted to hospital as a result of these ailments. Some conditions are more common in the severely obese, such as OSA, and such individuals may also present with trauma following road traffic accidents. Obtaining venous access can be difficult in morbidly obese patients, making a central line necessary. Airway management can also present problems due to a thick neck and more soft tissue.

Laparoscopic procedures also carry a higher risk of venous thromboembolism, and inflating the abdominal cavity with nitrogen during the procedure leads to compression of the vena cava and venous stasis. Thus, post-operatively there is an increased risk of pulmonary embolism in these patients. Lymphedema is more common and so also are problems such as cellulitis.

Patients with severe obesity admitted for any given medical condition are more likely to stay in hospital for longer compared to patients without obesity. They are also at higher risk of developing venous thromboembolism and pressure sores. Therefore, it is important to ensure that appropriate pressure relief mattresses are used and that thromboprophylaxis is prescribed for everyone unless contra-indicated.

Managing the severely obese in hospital

Hospitalization is an opportunity to discuss long-term plans for weight loss. Patients who have a severe illness may not wish to discuss weight loss. However, as patients are recovering from that illness, they may be more likely to engage with health professionals to try and lose weight to reduce further risk. This is especially relevant if their illness is a direct complication of their obesity. A good example would be a patient with obesity being diagnosed with T2DM following an admission with a myocardial infarction. Most of these patients would be highly motivated to lose weight to reduce future risk.

However, weight loss is often difficult to achieve, especially in patients with severe obesity. They are likely to have lost weight several times in the past and regained it. There may be difficulty with joint problems and inability to do adequate exercise. Depression is also common in this patient group, and there may be other psychological issues as well. Therefore, simply advising them to lose weight to reduce their disease risk may not be appropriate. Referral to weight management services following discharge is advised as often bariatric surgery may be required as a definitive procedure. Early referrals should be made to dieticians and physiotherapists to help start initiating weight loss and lifestyle changes.

Patient dignity is very important, and patients with severe obesity are entitled to the same respect from all hospital staff as any other patient in the hospital. All staff must be made aware that small comments that may be overheard by patients can be extremely distressing to the patient and damaging to their relationship with the health-care professionals trying to treat their illness. It is harder to care for patients with severe obesity from routine nursing care and drawing blood to the treatment of the very sick in intensive care. However, all staff should work together as a team to overcome this, and the hospital should invest in infrastructure and appliances so that the team can deliver the best care to all of their patients, even those with severe obesity.

Pitfalls

- Patients with morbid obesity often get admitted to hospital, but clinicians lose the opportunity to address weight as an issue with the patient.
- Identify needs for special hoists or beds prior to elective admissions.
- Be aware that there is a weight limit to a lot of hospital beds, CT or MRI scanners, operating theater tables, wheelchairs, and even weighing scales.
- Clinicians should highlight this need to the hospital management to ensure that care for the morbidly obese is not compromised as a result of inadequate equipment.

Key web links

American Society for Metabolic and Bariatric Surgery. http://asmbs.org/ [accessed on December 29, 2012].
Weight control Information Network (WIN). http://win.niddk.nih.gov/publications/medical.htm#optimal [accessed on December 29, 2012].
http://win.niddk.nih.gov/publications/PDFs/medcareobesebw.pdf [accessed on December 29, 2012].

Further reading

Adams, J.P. & Murphy, P.G. (2000) Obesity in anaesthesia and intensive care. *British Journal of Anaesthesia*, 85, 91–108.
Folmann, N.B., Bossen, K.S., Willaing, I. *et al.* (2007) Obesity, hospital services use and costs. *Advances in Health Economics and Health Services Research*, 17, 319–332.

Geary, B. & Collins, N. (2011) Are we prepared for a growing population? Morbid obesity and its implications in Irish emergency departments. *European Journal of Emergency Medicine*, 19, 271–274.

National Task Force on the Prevention and Treatment of Obesity. (2002) Medical care for obese patients: advice for health care professionals. *American Family Physician*, 65, 81–88.

Conversion Table

Measurement	Convert from metric or SI units to conventional	Convert from conventional to metric or SI units
Body mass index (BMI) kg/m²		(pounds/inches²) × 703
Height and circumference	cm = 0.394 inches	Inches = 2.54 cm
Weight	kg = 2.2 pounds	Pound = 0.45 kg
Energy	kJ = kcal/4.18	kcal = 4.18 kJ
Distance	km = 0.62 miles	Mile = 1.61 km
Volume	mL = 0.034 ounces	Ounce = 29.6 mL
Glucose	mmol/L = 0.055 × mg/dL	mg/dL = 18.02 × mmol/L
Cholesterol	mmol/L = mg/dL/38.7	mg/dL = 38.7 × mmol/L
Triglycerides	mmol/L = mg/dL/88.6	mg/dL = 88.6 × mmol/L

Practical Manual of Clinical Obesity, First Edition. Robert Kushner, Victor Lawrence and Sudhesh Kumar.
© 2013 John Wiley & Sons, Ltd. Published 2013 by John Wiley & Sons, Ltd.

Index

Practical Manual of Clinical Obesity, First Edition. Robert Kushner, Victor Lawrence
and Sudhesh Kumar.
© 2013 John Wiley & Sons, Ltd. Published 2013 by John Wiley & Sons, Ltd.

Printed and bound by CPI Group (UK) Ltd, Croydon, CR0 4YY

27/10/2024

14580144-0003

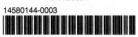